FAT AND SKINNY

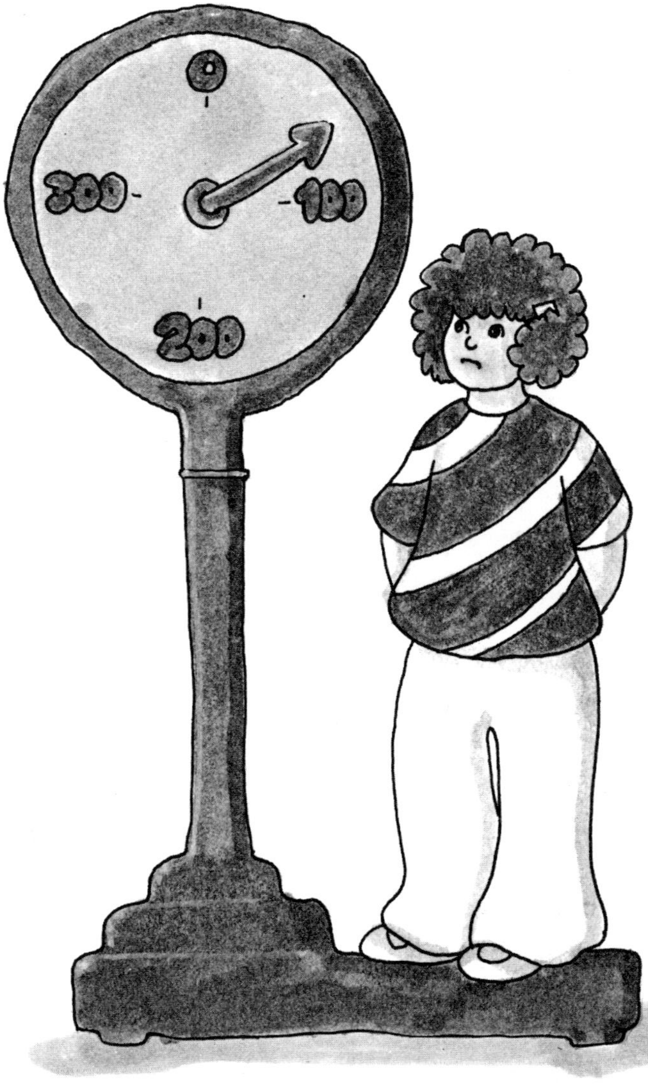

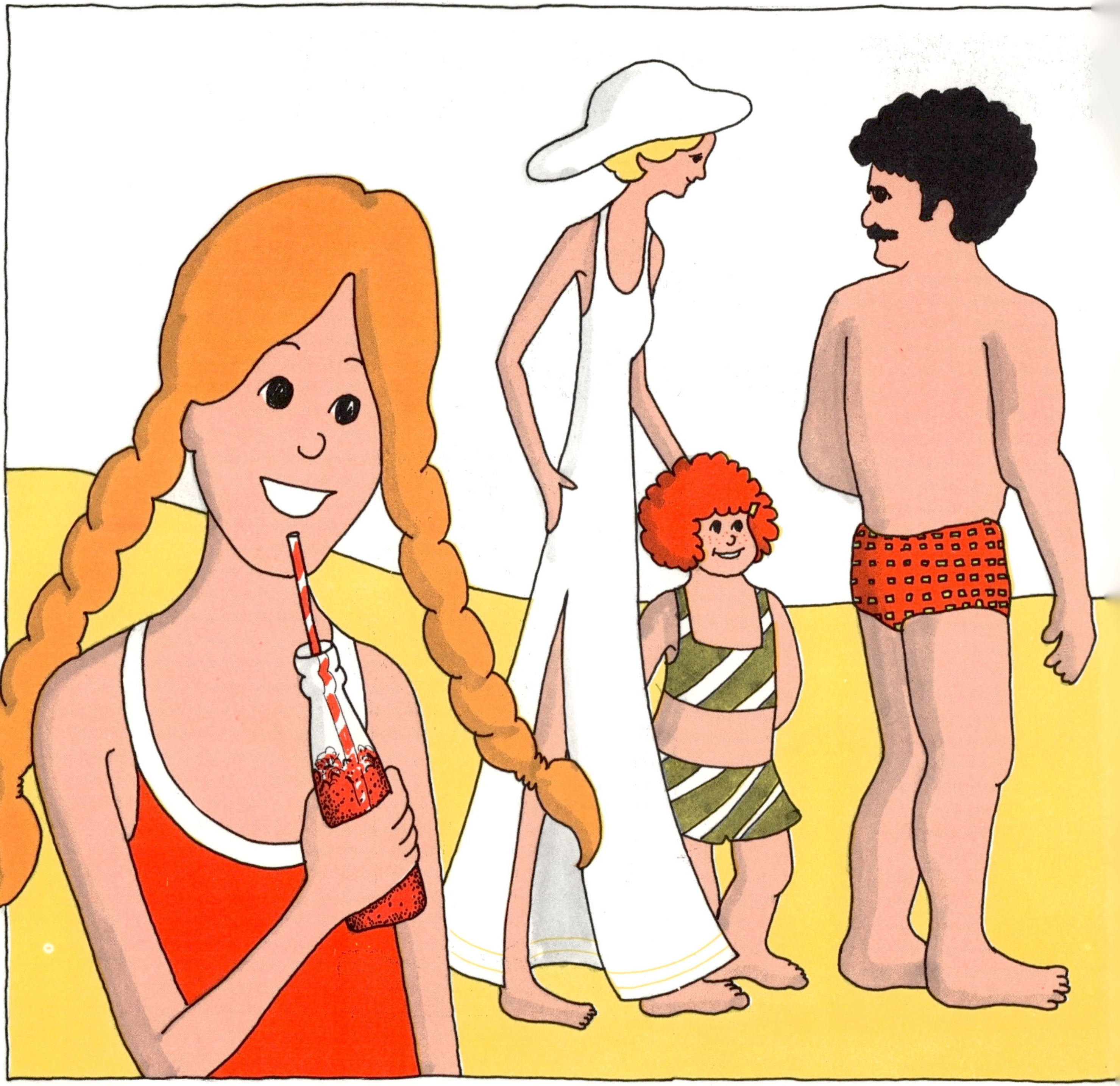

FAT AND SKINNY

By Philip Balestrino   Illustrated by Pam Makie

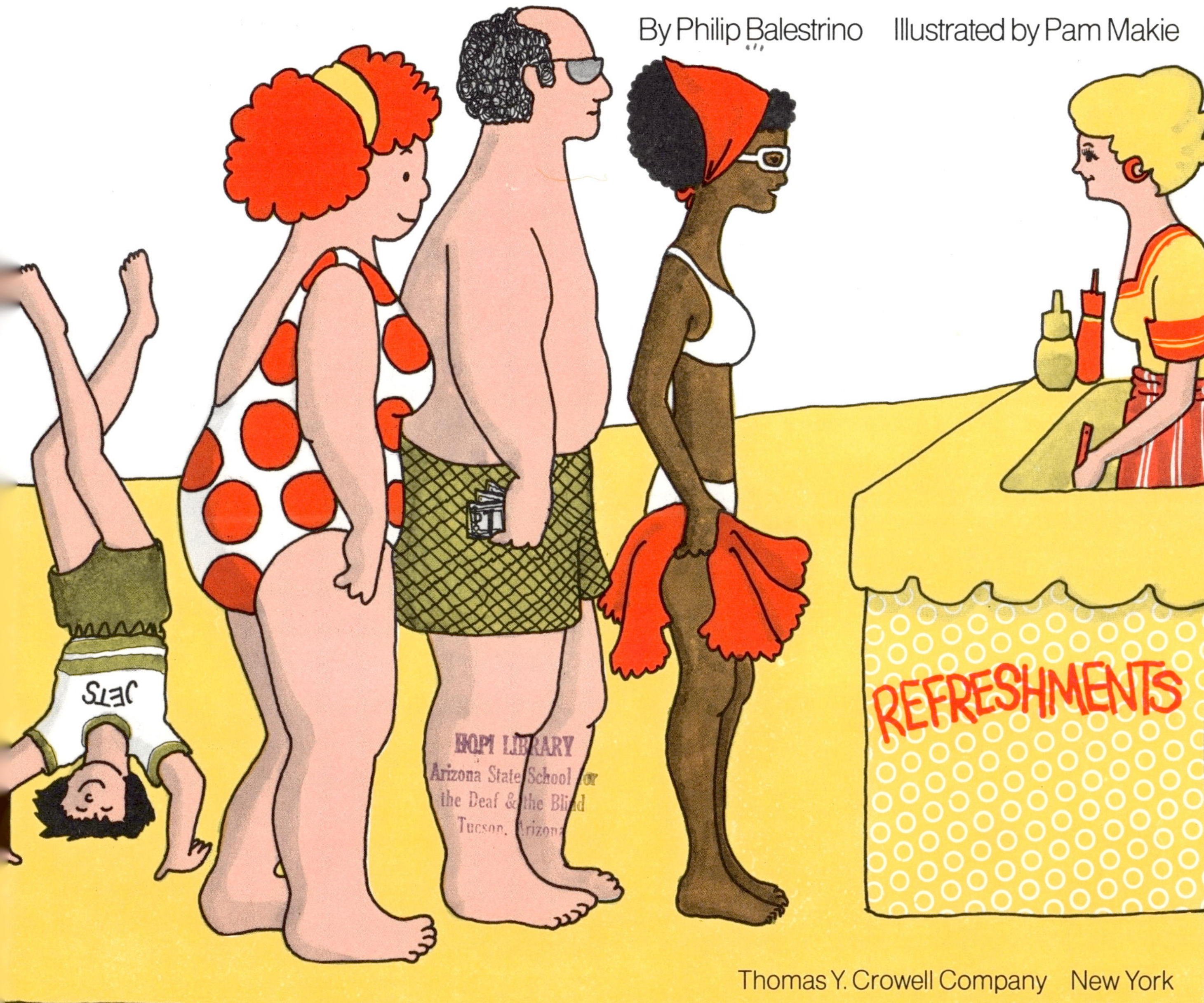

Thomas Y. Crowell Company   New York

LET'S-READ-AND-FIND-OUT SCIENCE BOOKS

LIVING THINGS: PLANTS

Down Come the Leaves
How a Seed Grows
Mushrooms and Molds
Plants in Winter
Seeds by Wind and Water
The Sunlit Sea
A Tree Is a Plant
Where Does Your Garden Grow?

LIVING THINGS: ANIMALS, BIRDS, FISH, INSECTS, ETC.

Animals in Winter
Bats in the Dark
Bees and Beelines
Big Tracks, Little Tracks
Birds at Night
Birds Eat and Eat and Eat
Bird Talk
The Blue Whale
Camels: Ships of the Desert
Cockroaches: Here, There, and Everywhere
Ducks Don't Get Wet
The Emperor Penguins
Fireflies in the Night
Giraffes at Home
Green Grass and White Milk
Green Turtle Mysteries
Hummingbirds in the Garden
Hungry Sharks
It's Nesting Time
Ladybug, Ladybug, Fly Away Home
The Long-Lost Coelacanth and Other Living Fossils
My Daddy Longlegs
My Visit to the Dinosaurs
Opossum
Sandpipers
Shrimps
Spider Silk
Spring Peepers
Starfish
Twist, Wiggle, and Squirm: A Book About Earthworms
Watch Honeybees with Me
What I Like About Toads
Why Frogs Are Wet

THE HUMAN BODY

A Baby Starts to Grow
Before You Were a Baby
A Drop of Blood
Fat and Skinny
Find Out by Touching
Follow Your Nose
Hear Your Heart
How Many Teeth?
How You Talk
In the Night
*Look at Your Eyes**
My Five Senses
My Hands
The Skeleton Inside You
Sleep Is for Everyone
*Straight Hair, Curly Hair**
Use Your Brain
What Happens to a Hamburger
*Your Skin and Mine**

And other books on AIR, WATER, AND WEATHER; THE EARTH AND ITS COMPOSITION; ASTRONOMY AND SPACE; and MATTER AND ENERGY

**Available in Spanish*

Library of Congress Cataloging in Publication Data Balestrino, Philip. Fat and skinny. (Let's-read-and-find-out science books) SUMMARY: Briefly explains how metabolism affects how fat or skinny a person is. 1. Metabolism—Juv. lit. [1. Metabolism] I. Makie, Pam, illus. II. Title. QP171.B315 1975 612'.39 74-12306 ISBN 0-690-00454-0 ISBN 0-690-00665-9 (lib. bdg).

1 2 3 4 5 6 7 8 9 10

FAT AND SKINNY

LET'S READ AND FIND OUT

People may be short and skinny, or short and fat. They may be tall and skinny, or tall and fat. People may have long fingers or short, thick fingers or thin. They may have big fat bellies, or thin flat bellies. They may have big feet or little feet, big ears or little ears, blue eyes or brown. People are different.

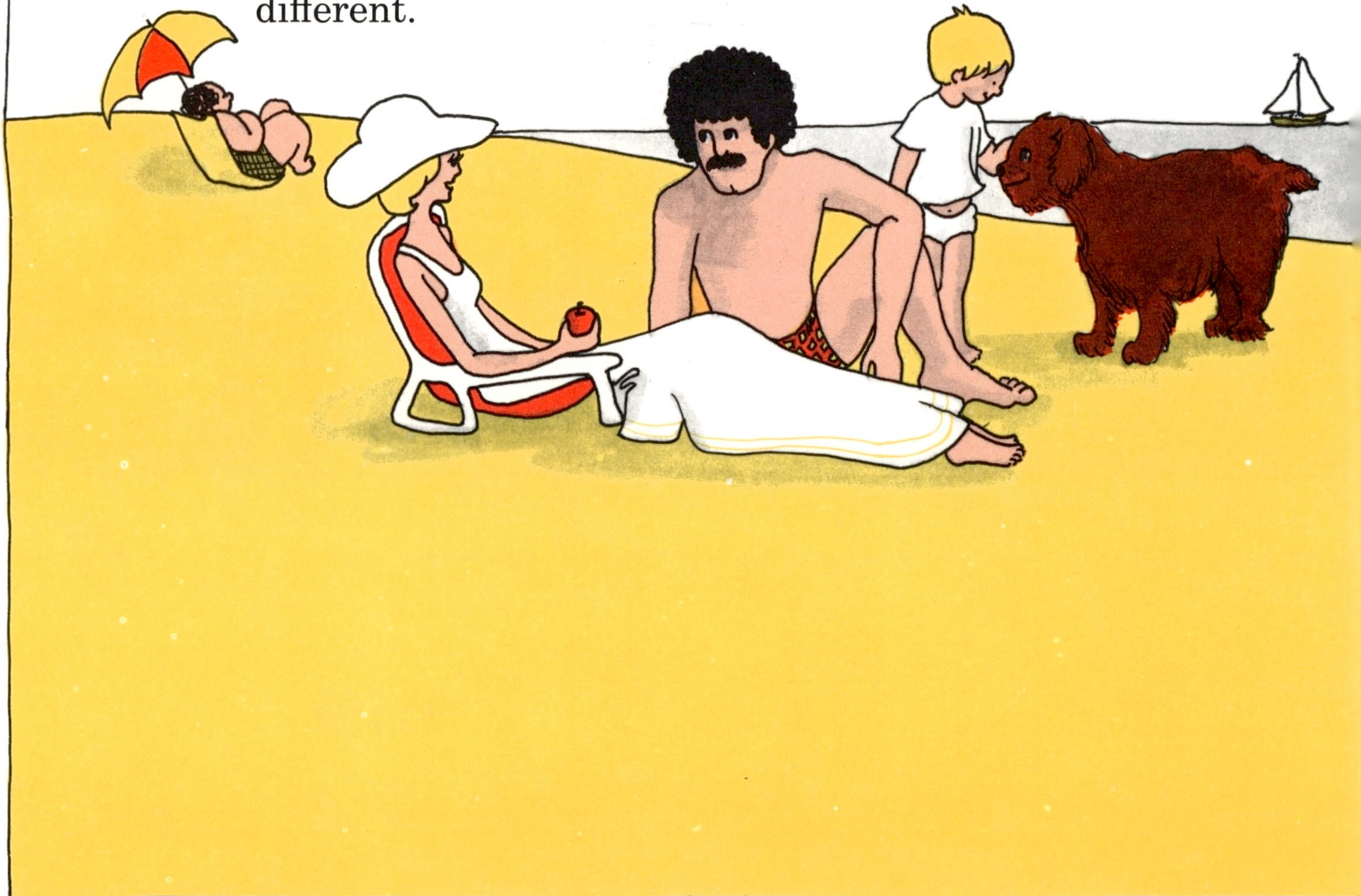

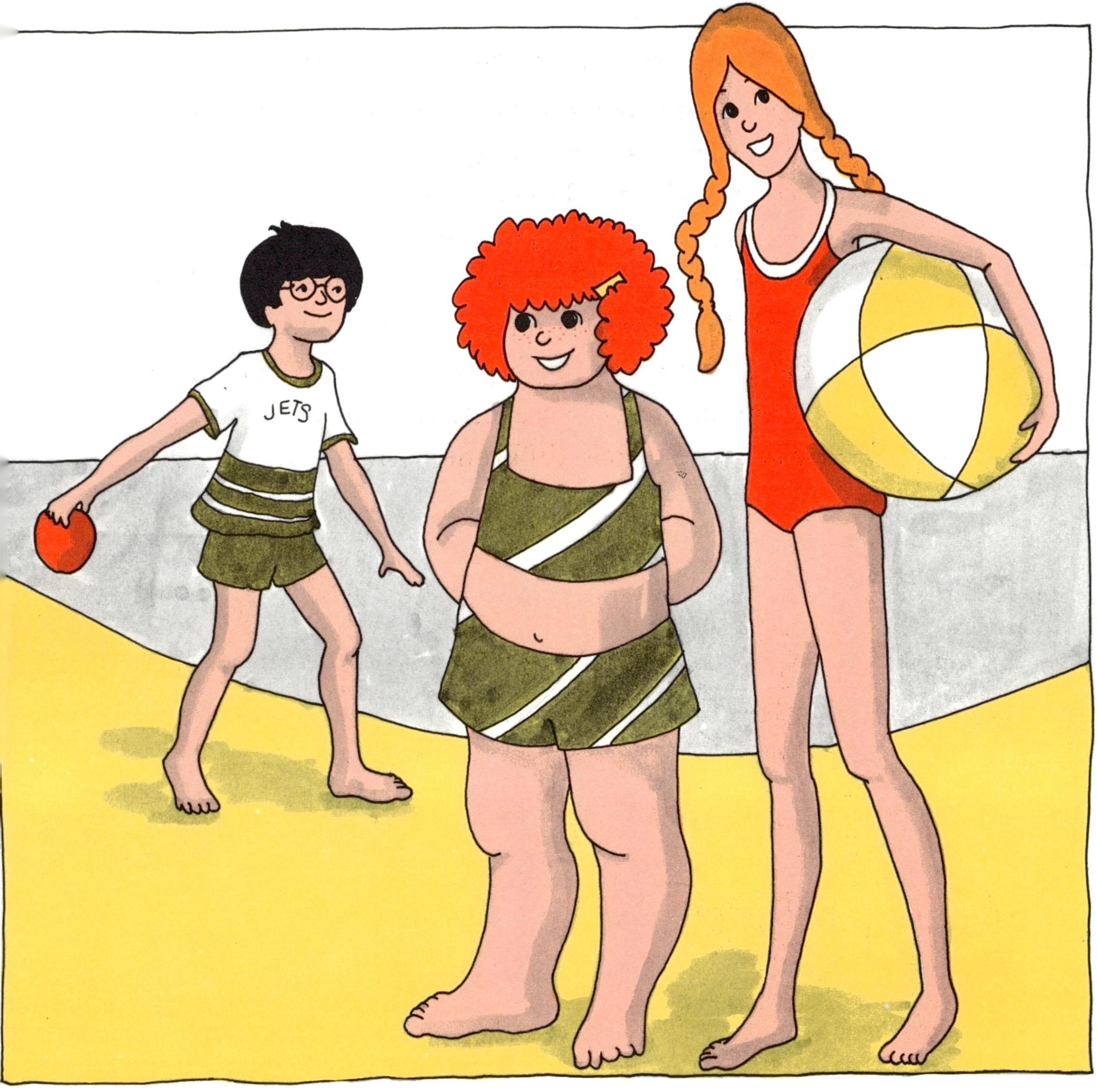
JETS

They eat different foods and they do different things. Some people play more than they sleep. Some sleep more than they play. Some like chocolate cake for dessert, others like apples. Some people are fat, and some are skinny. Some are in between. But everybody, even a very skinny person, has some fat on his body.

Fat is good for you. It gives shape to your body. Your hands, ears, toes, legs, and arms—every part of you—would look different without fat.

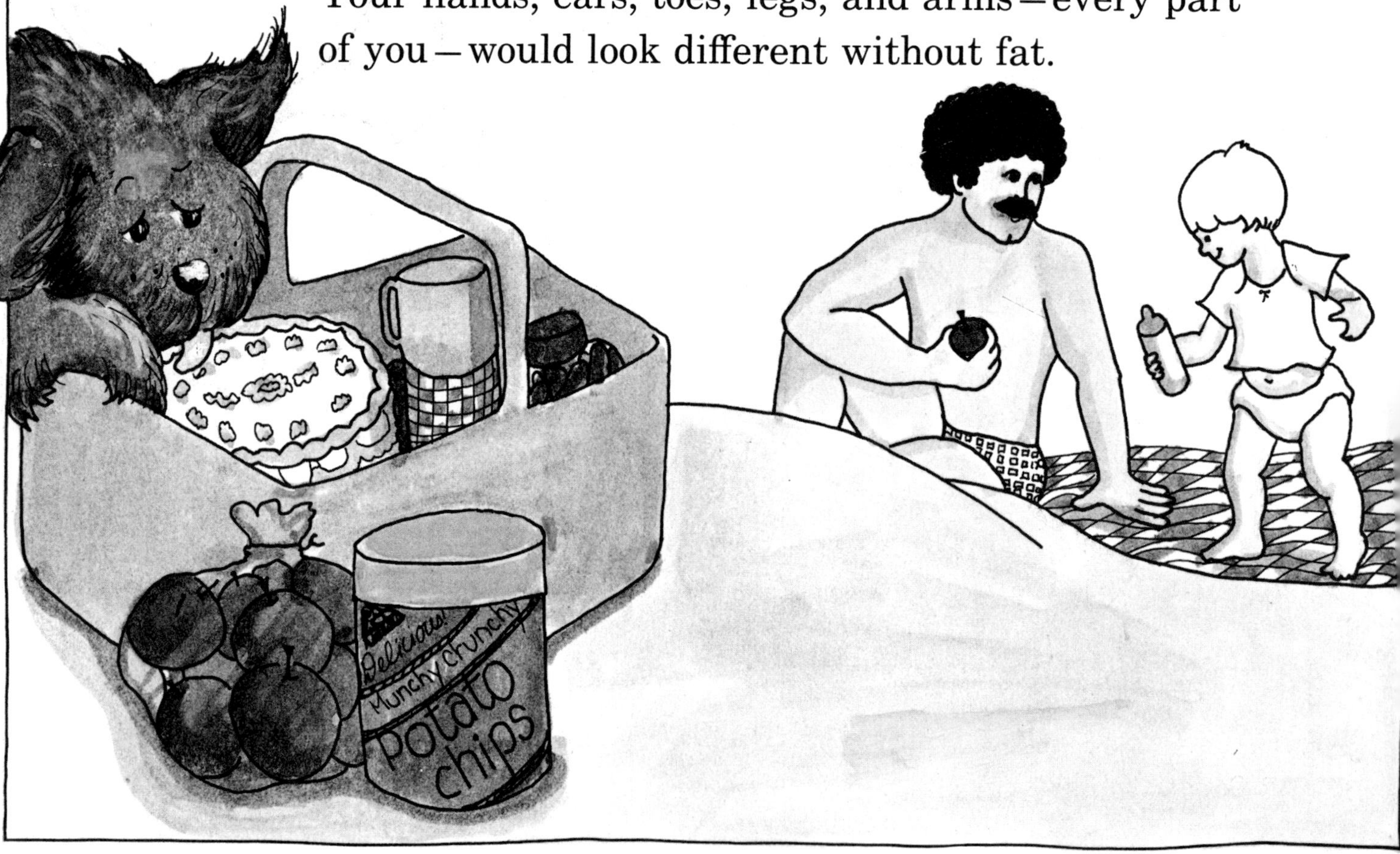

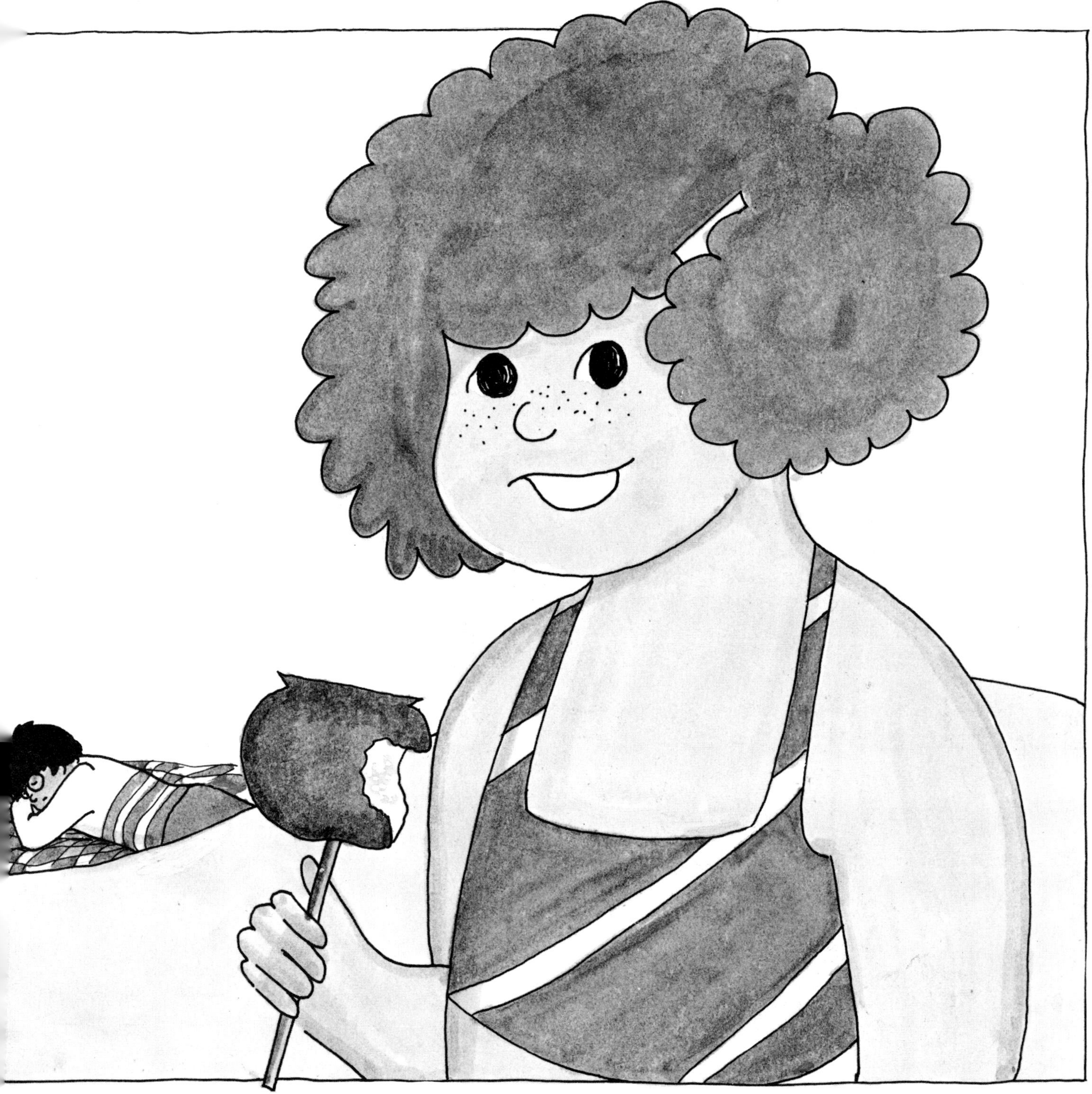

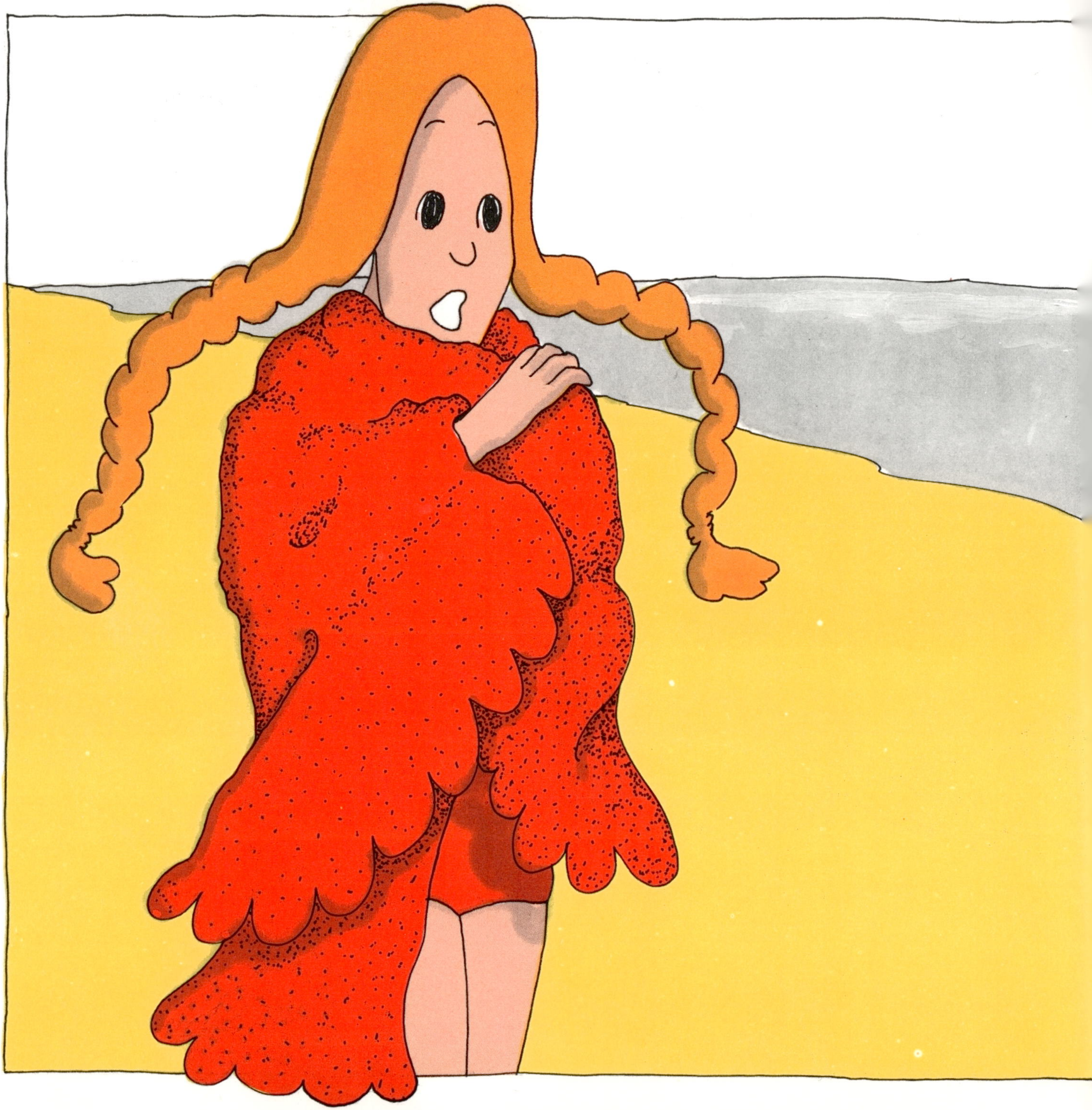

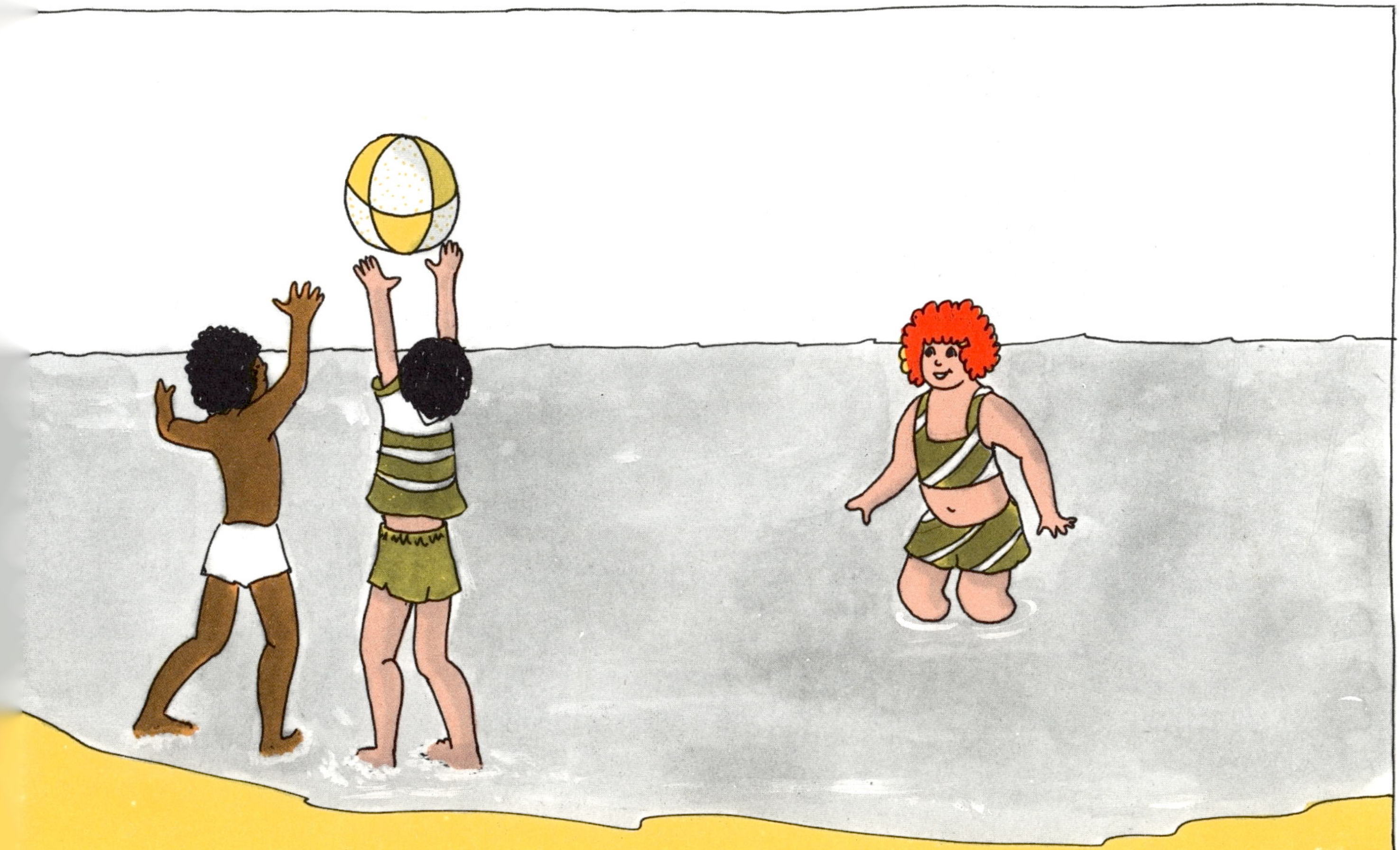

Fat also keeps you warm. In winter your hands, feet, nose, and neck get cold because they have less fat than the rest of you. Fat people need less clothing than thin people. The extra fat acts like an overcoat to keep them warm. In the water at the beach, fat people don't shiver as much as skinny people. The fat keeps them warm.

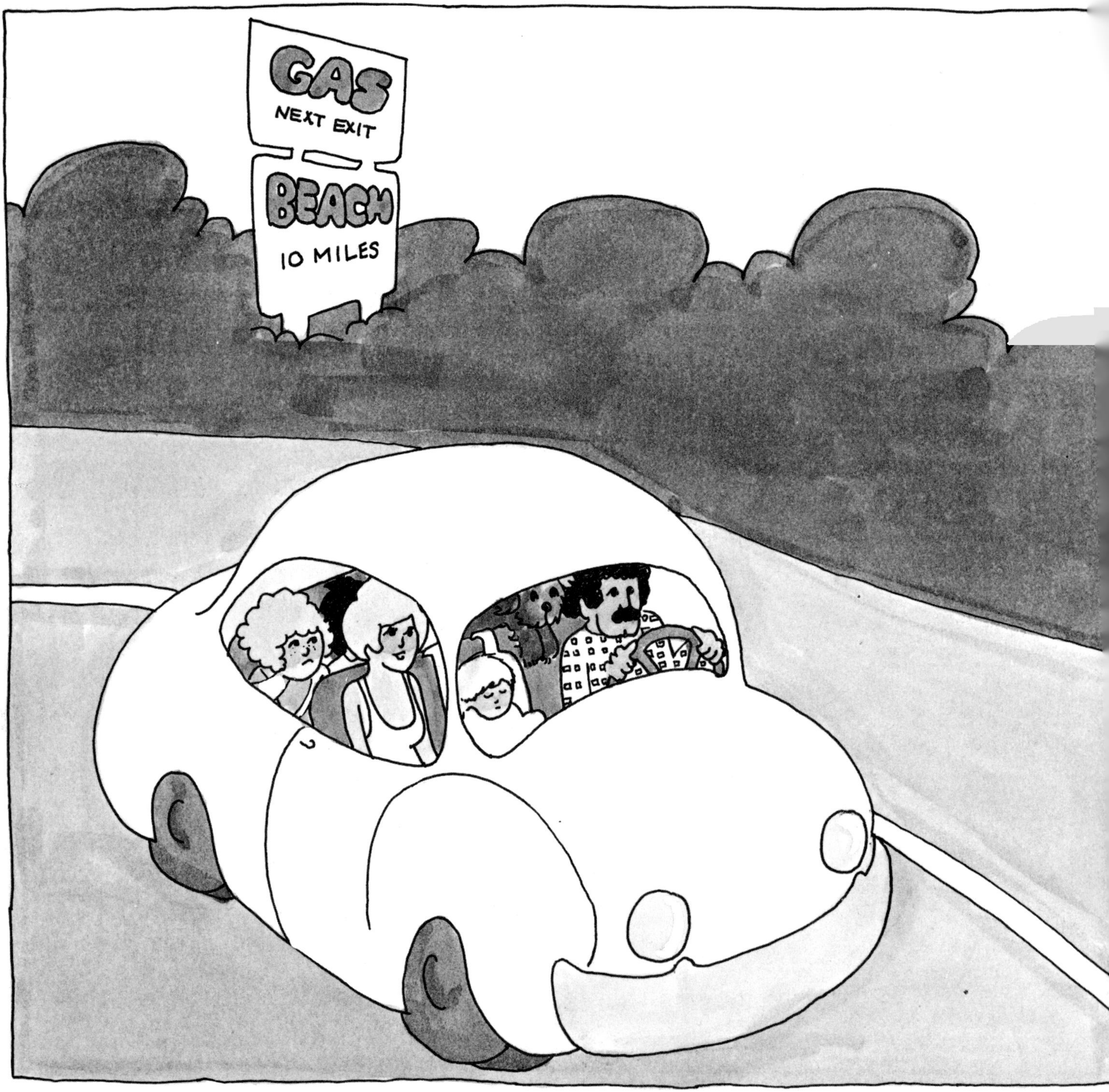
GAS
NEXT EXIT
BEACH
10 MILES

Fat is used by your body to make heat. Fat is fuel for your body, the way gasoline is fuel for a car or truck. A truck with a heavy load uses more fuel than an empty truck. If the truck isn't moving, very little fuel is needed to keep the motor running. People who move a lot use more fuel than people who don't.

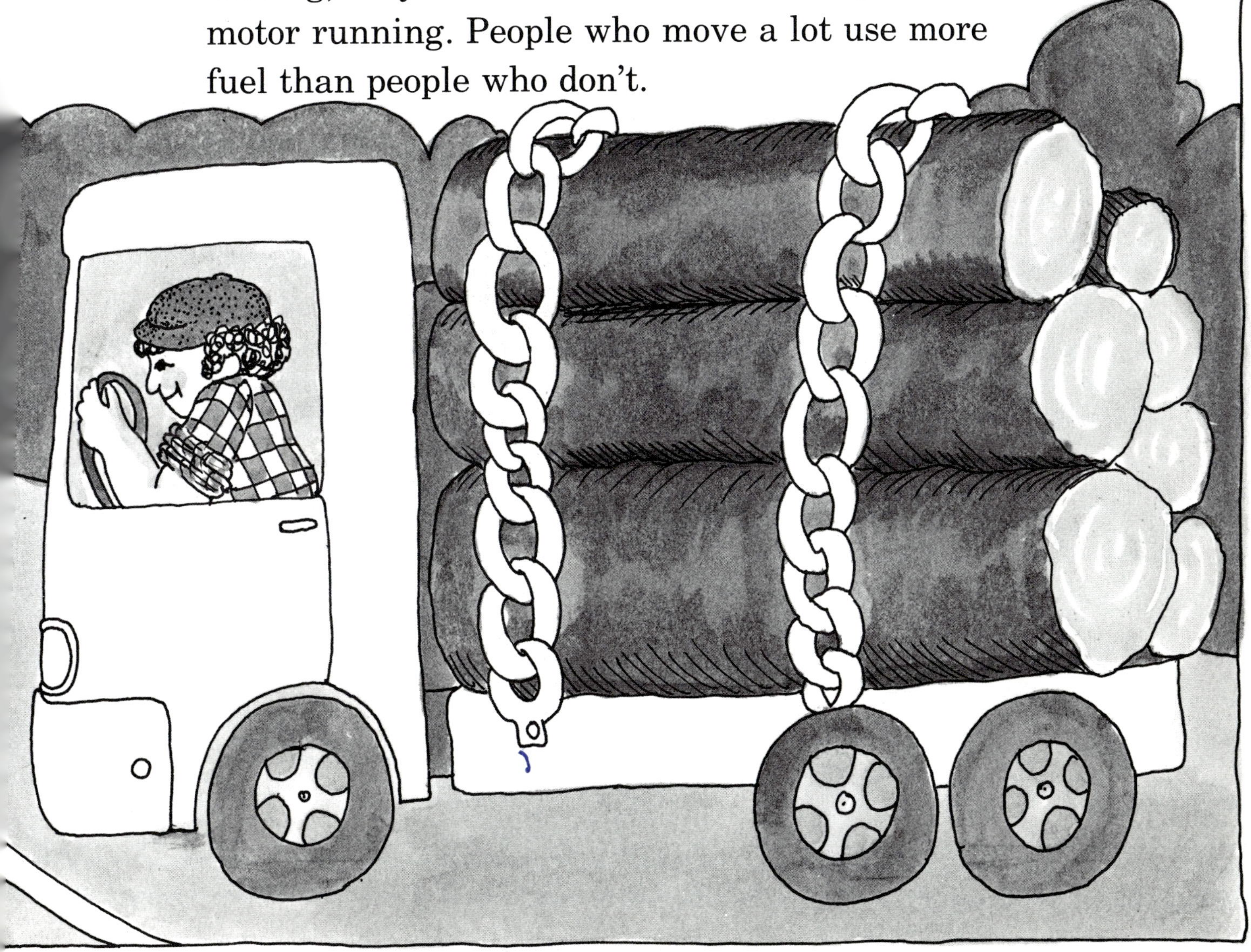

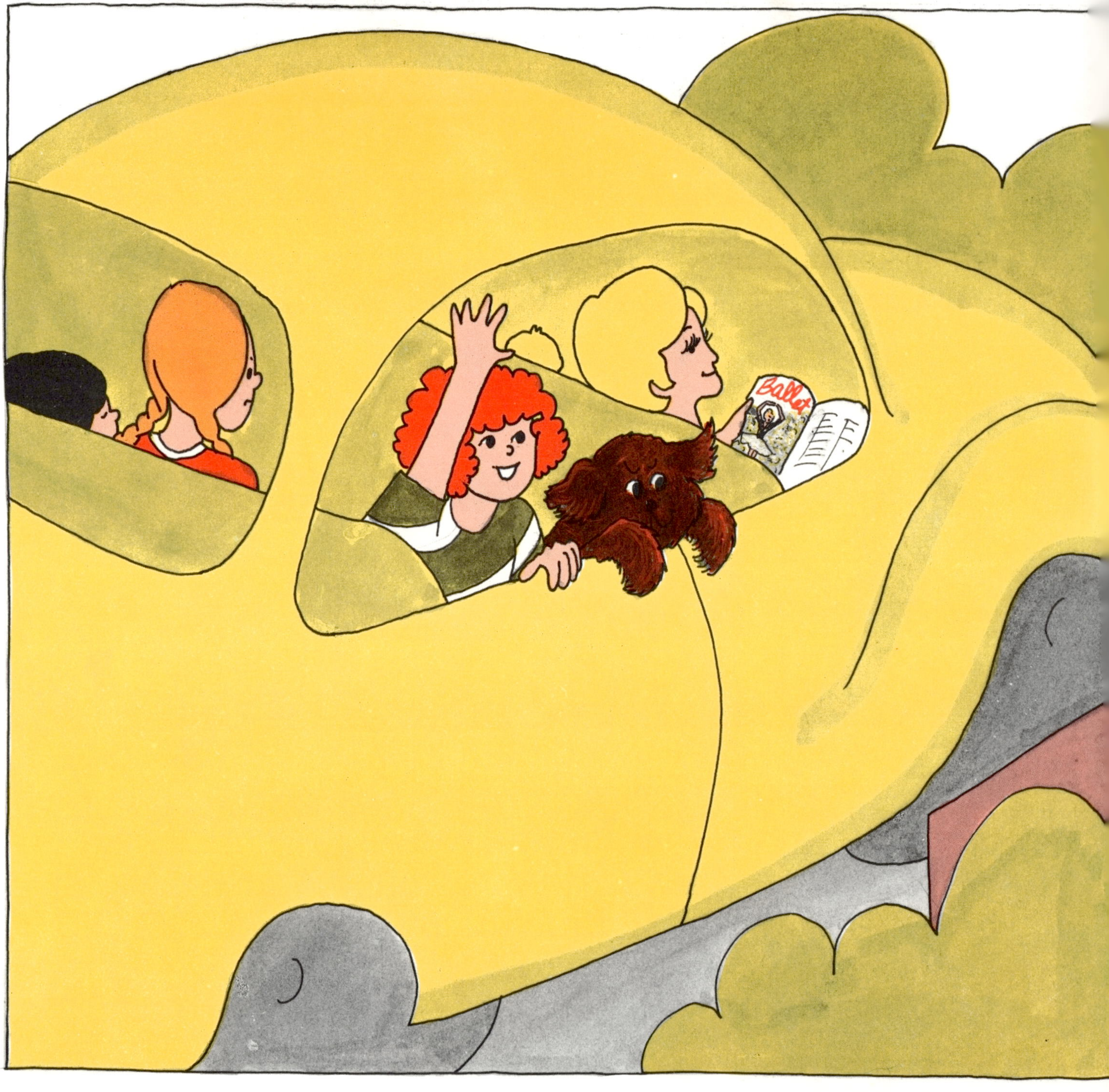
Ballet

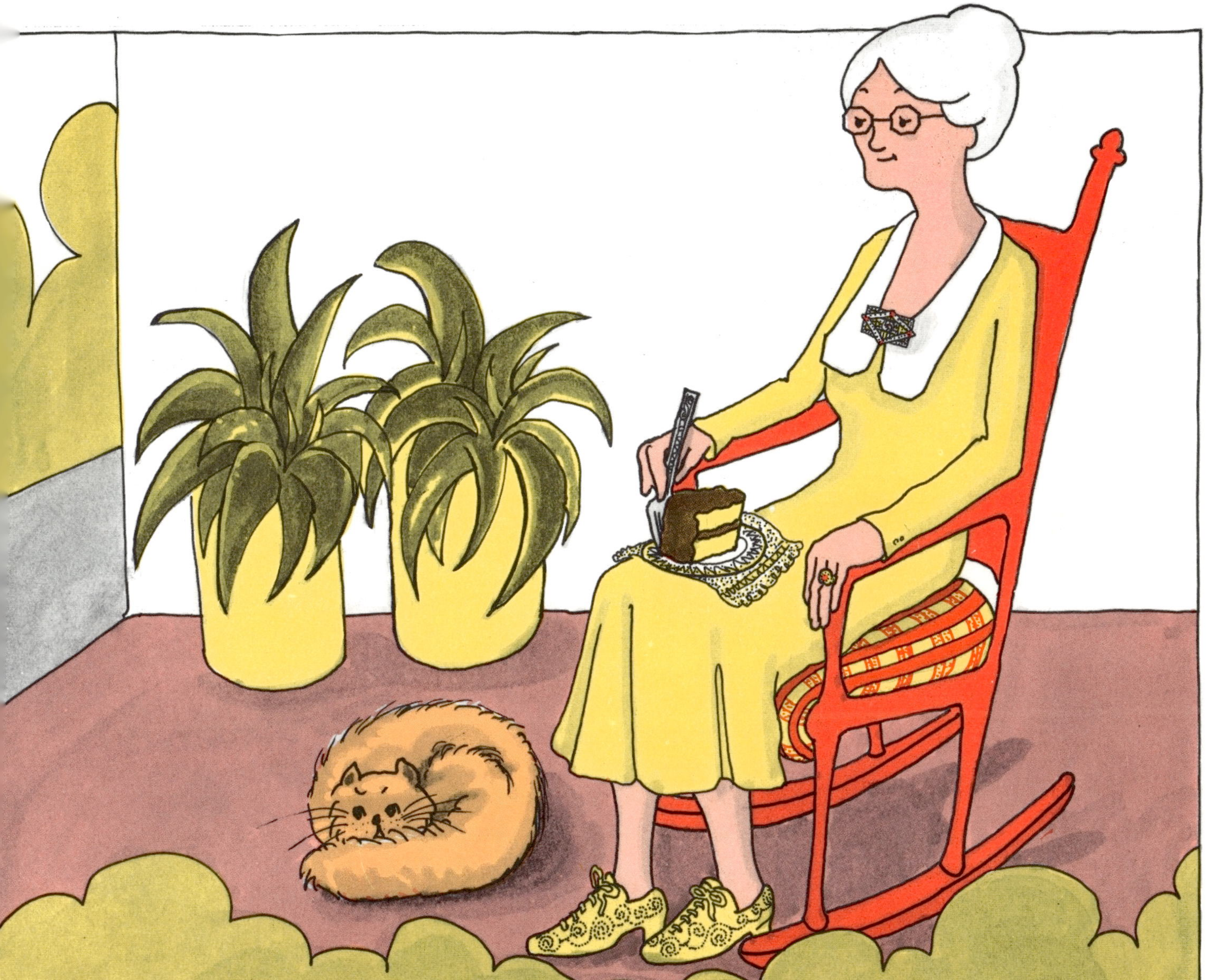

Dancers move a lot, so they use a lot of fuel. Artists and teachers don't move as much, so they don't use as much fuel. An old lady who sits all day needs fuel, too—just to keep warm.

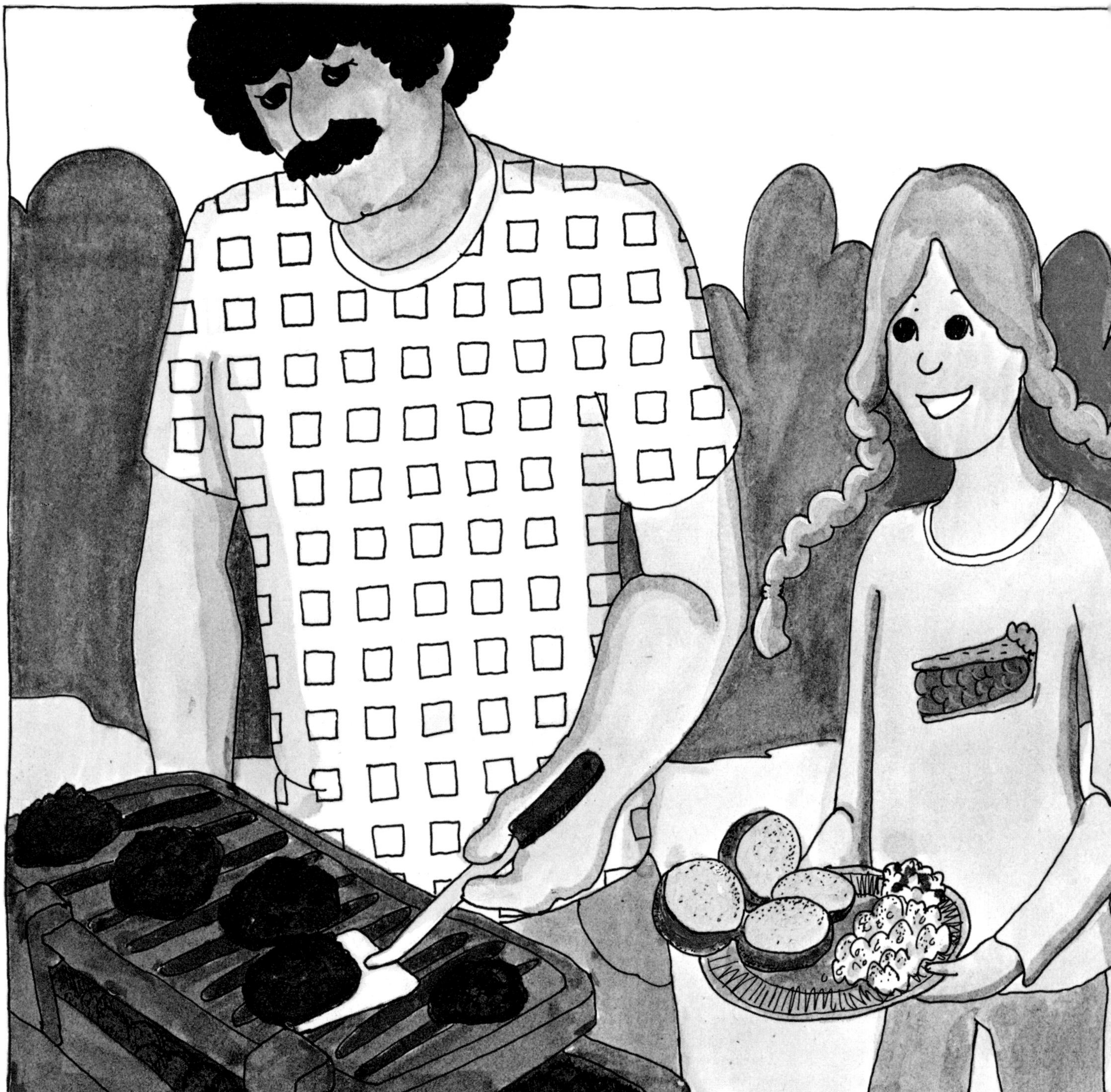

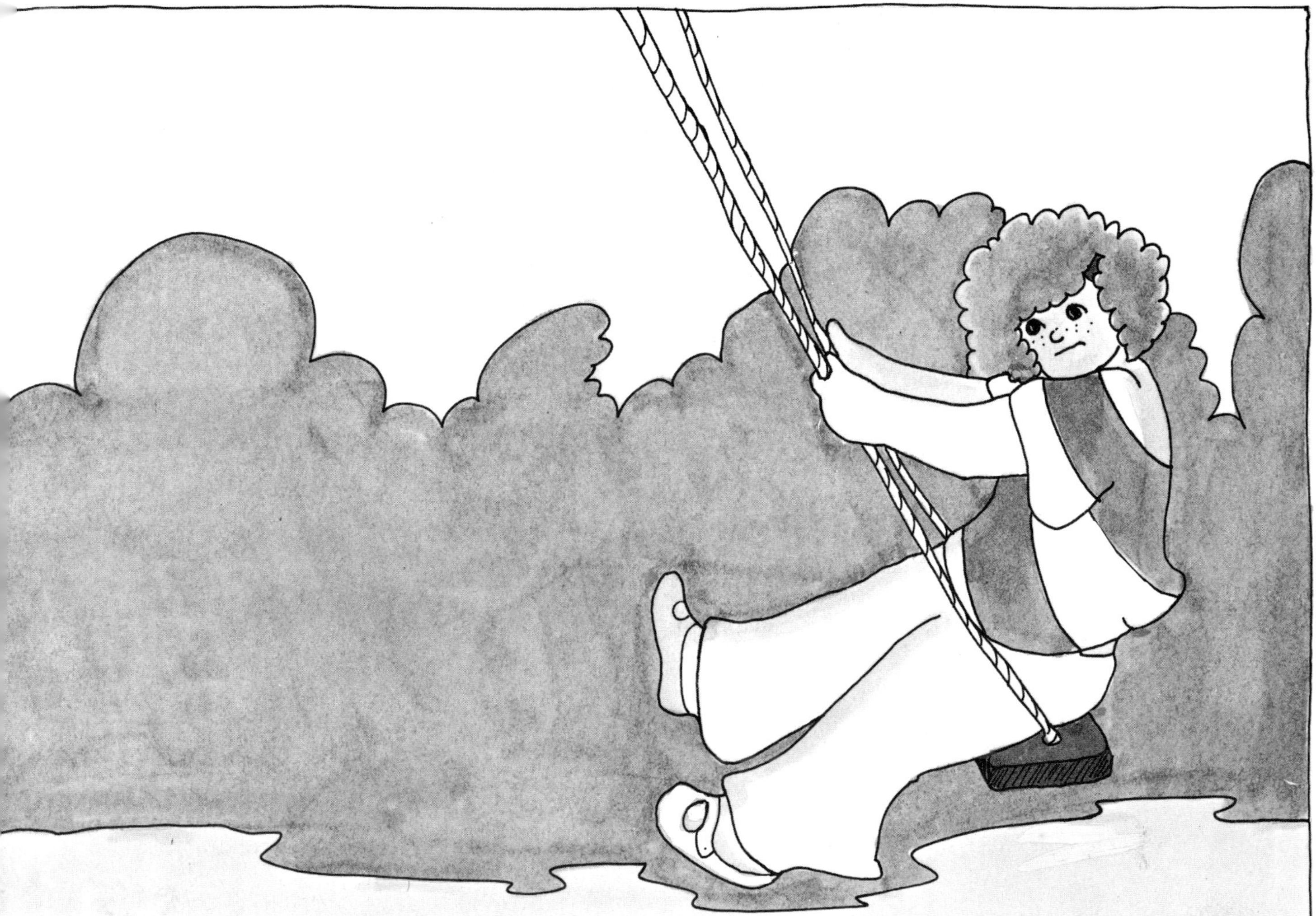

Some skinny people who want to get fat eat a lot of food. But they may never get fat.

Some fat people who want to get thin eat less food. But they may not get much thinner.

That's because of metabolism.

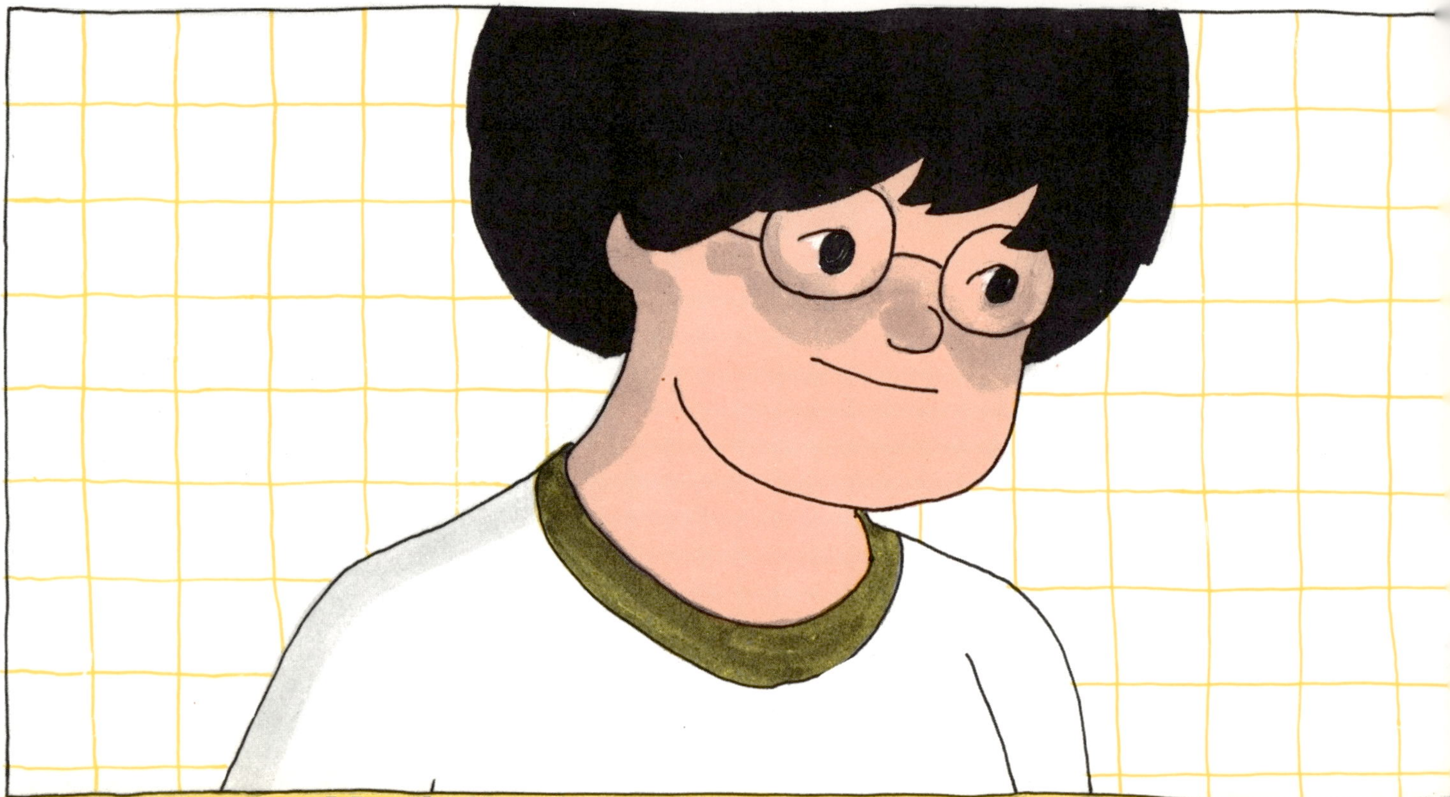

Metabolism means change—how a person changes food to fat, and how he uses the fat that is stored in his body. Some people burn up food faster than others. How fast the food is turned into energy is known as the rate of metabolism. Some people have high metabolism. That means they use food fast. Many thin people have high metabolism. Other people have low metabolism. That means they store food in their bodies, and use it slowly. Many fat people have low metabolism.

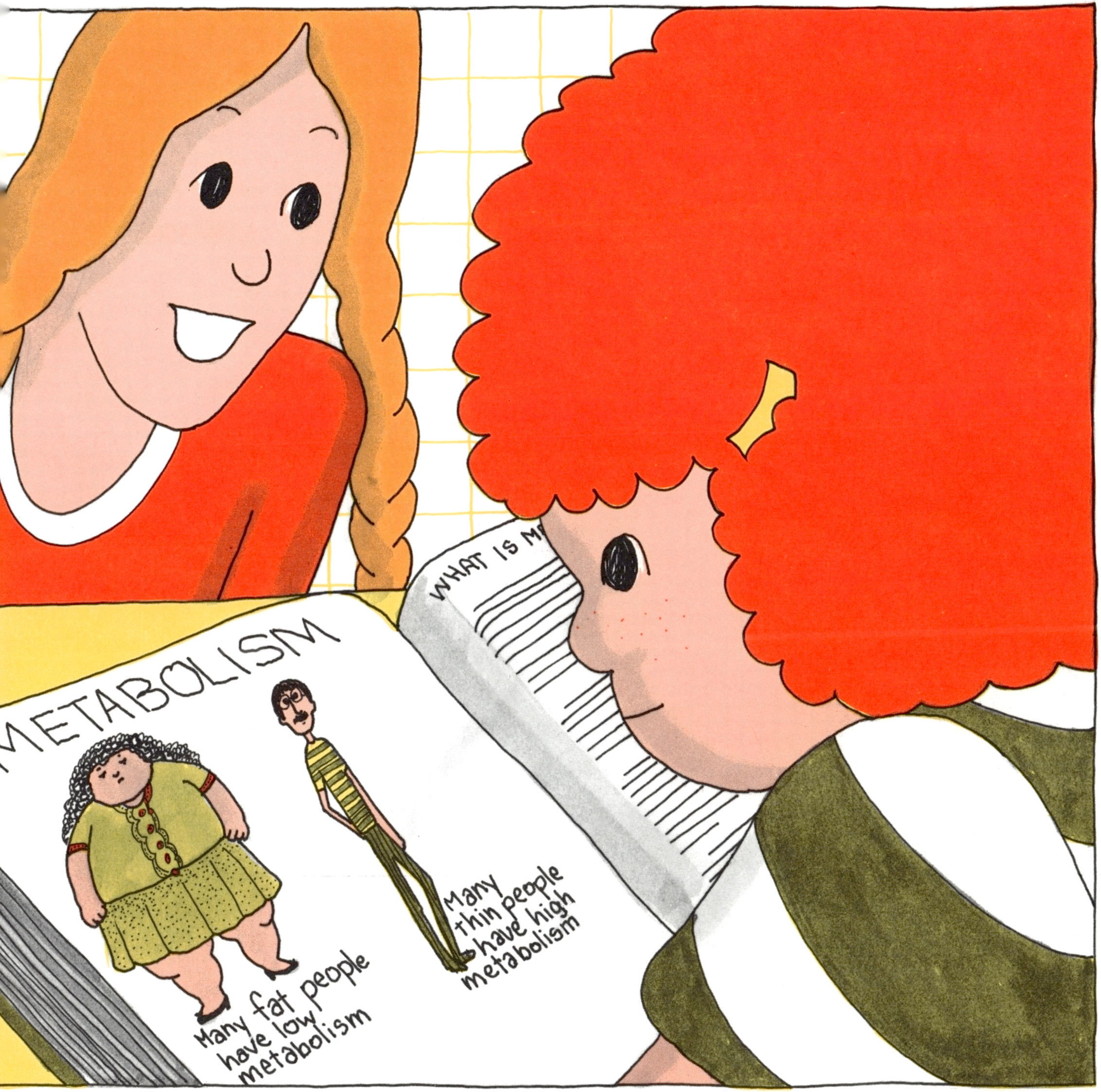
METABOLISM
Many fat people have low metabolism
Many thin people have high metabolism
WHAT IS M

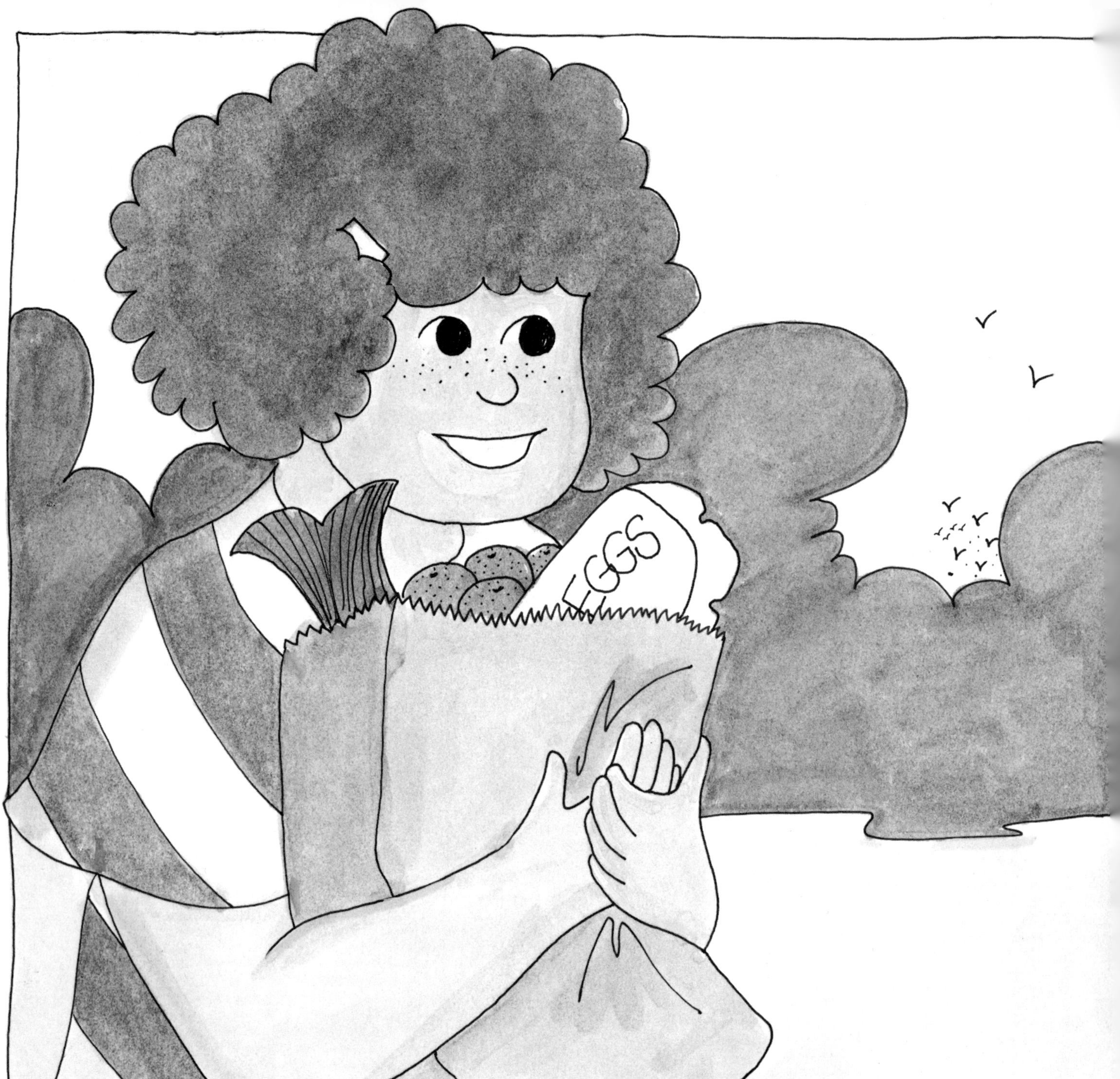
EGGS

The rate of metabolism does not depend on how much food is eaten by a person. A fat person can usually raise his metabolism by exercising more and by eating such food as meat, chicken, fish, and eggs.

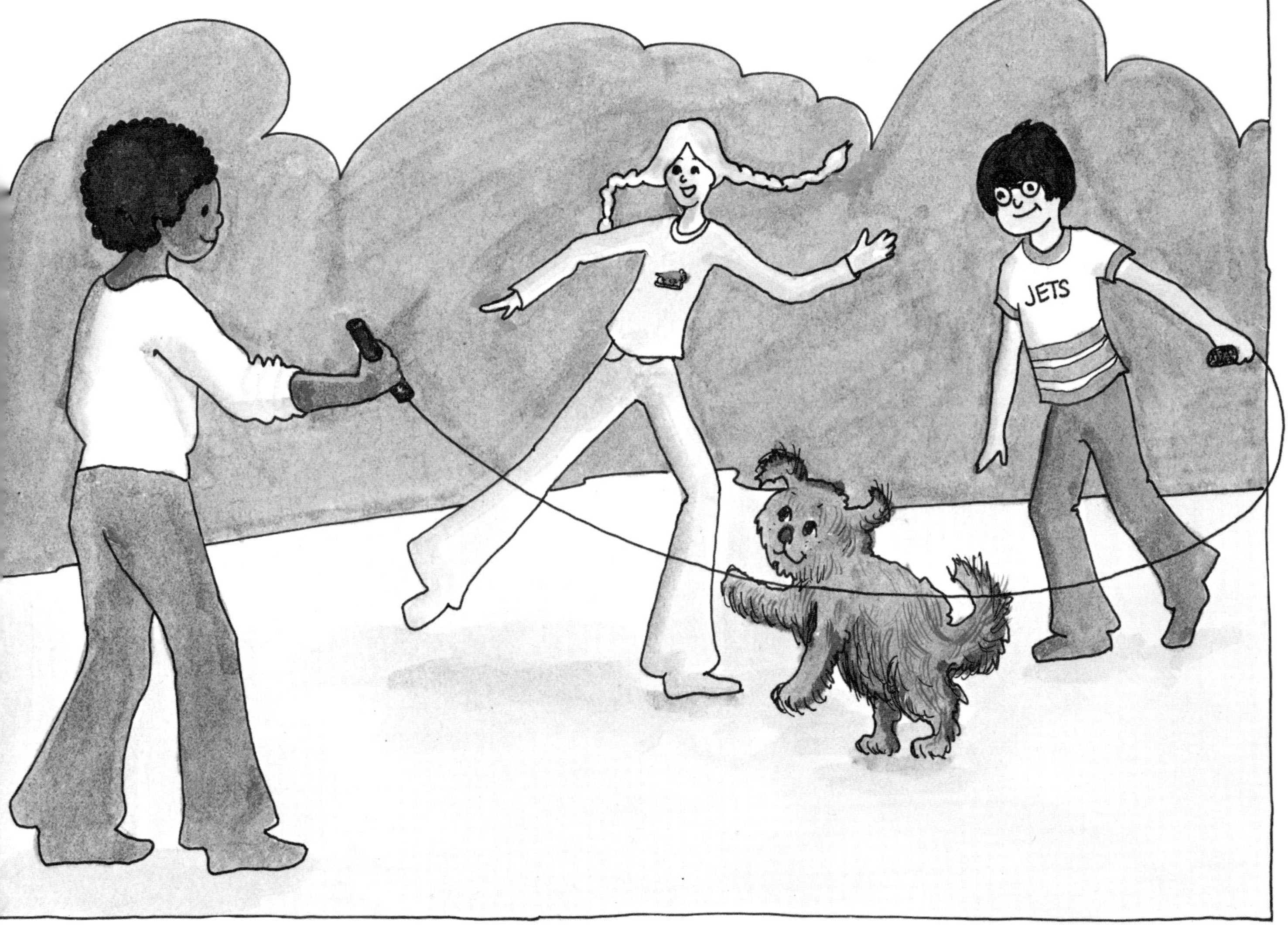

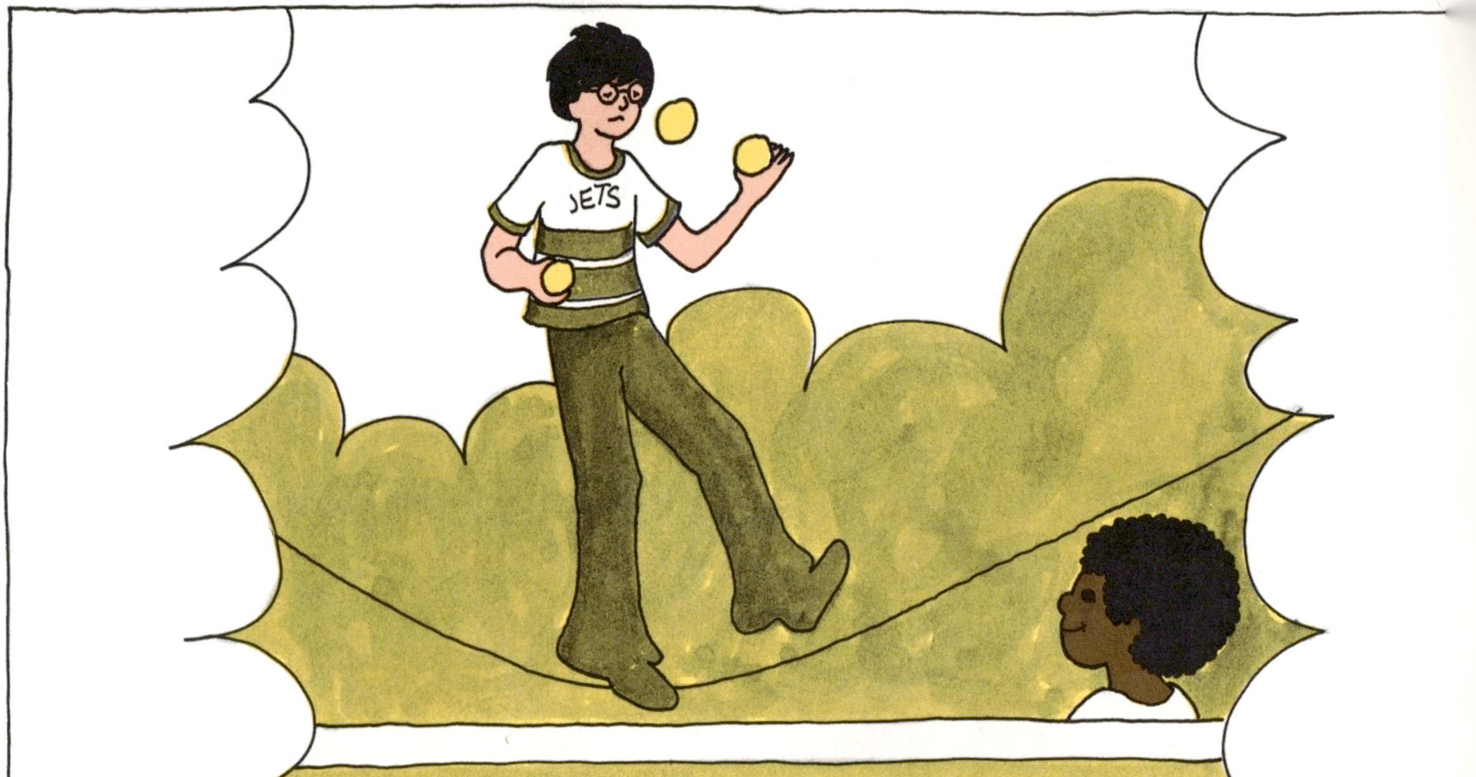

A skinny person might eat more than a fat person. The skinny person might run and jump and play a lot. The fat person might move more slowly. He might like to sit and eat. And he might eat cake and pie, ice cream and doughnuts, piles of potatoes and gravy. These foods have lots of calories. Calories are the way we measure the amount of energy each food will become. Some foods make more energy than others. We say they have more calories.

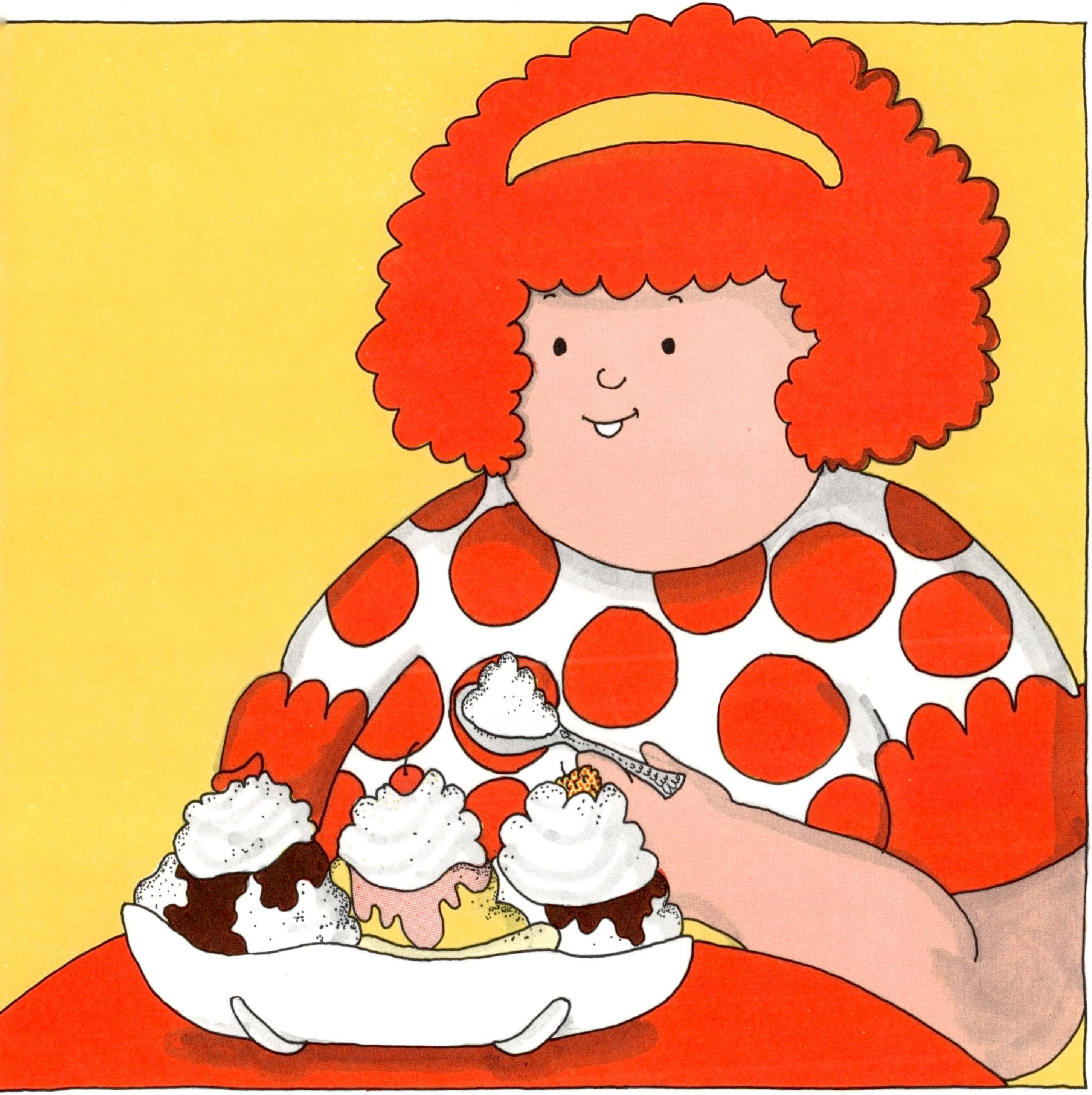

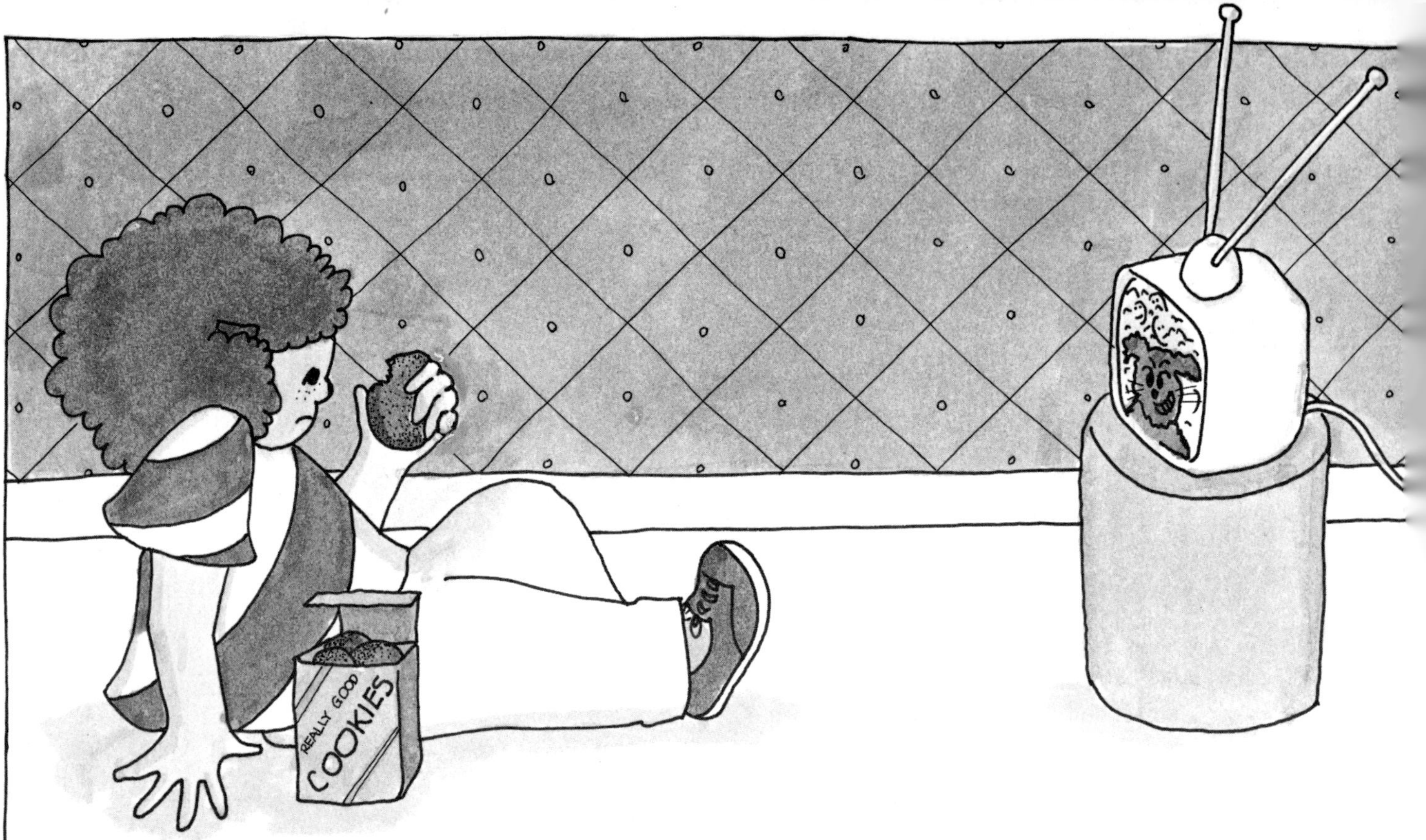

Carrots and beans, apples and oranges, don't have as many calories as some other foods.

If a person eats a pound of cookies and watches television all day, he doesn't use up the calories. He is not using the fuel, so his body stores it away. If he doesn't run and play and use up the stored food, it will probably stay in his body as fat. The more he eats, the more fuel he stores away, and the fatter he becomes.

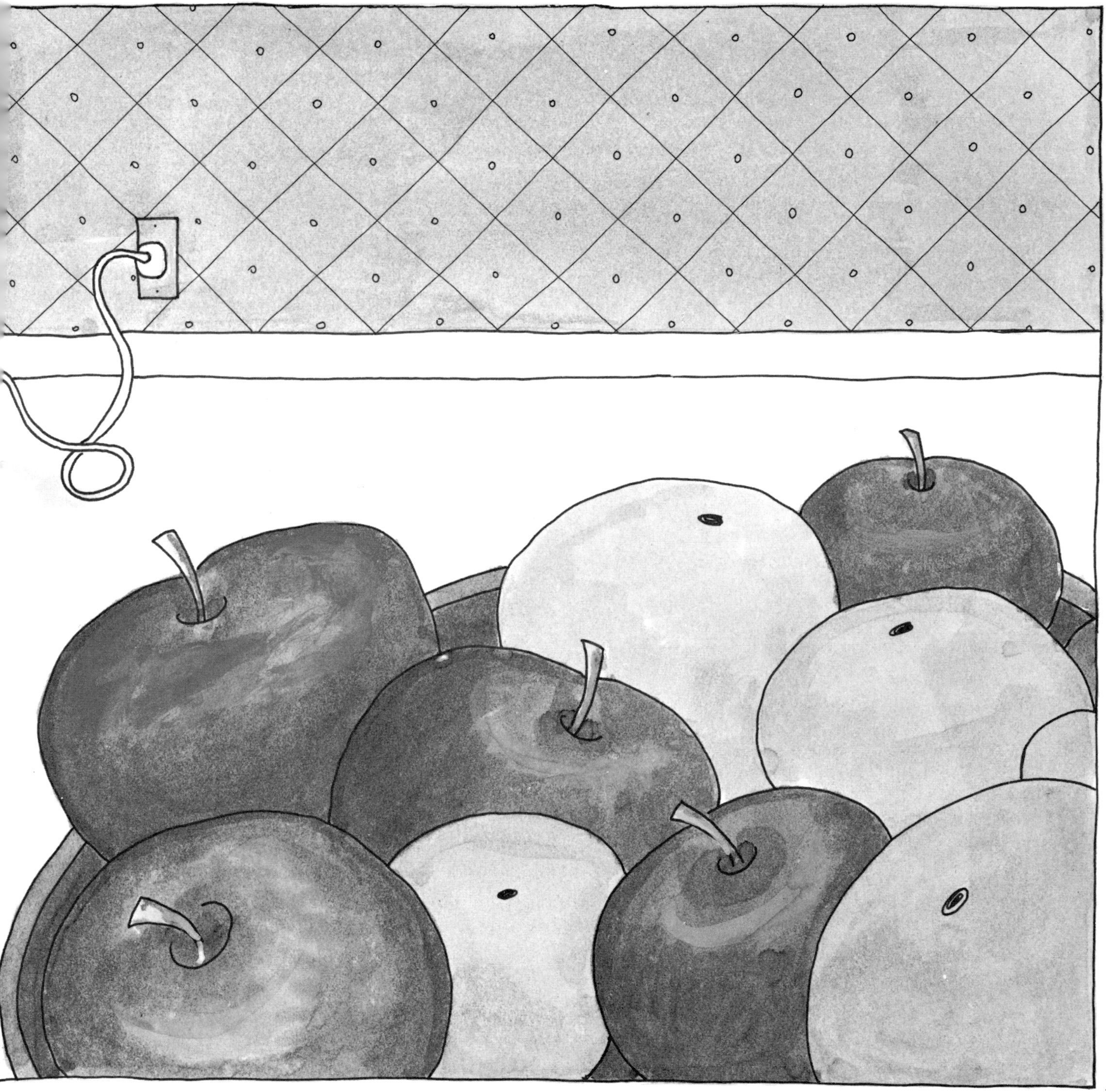

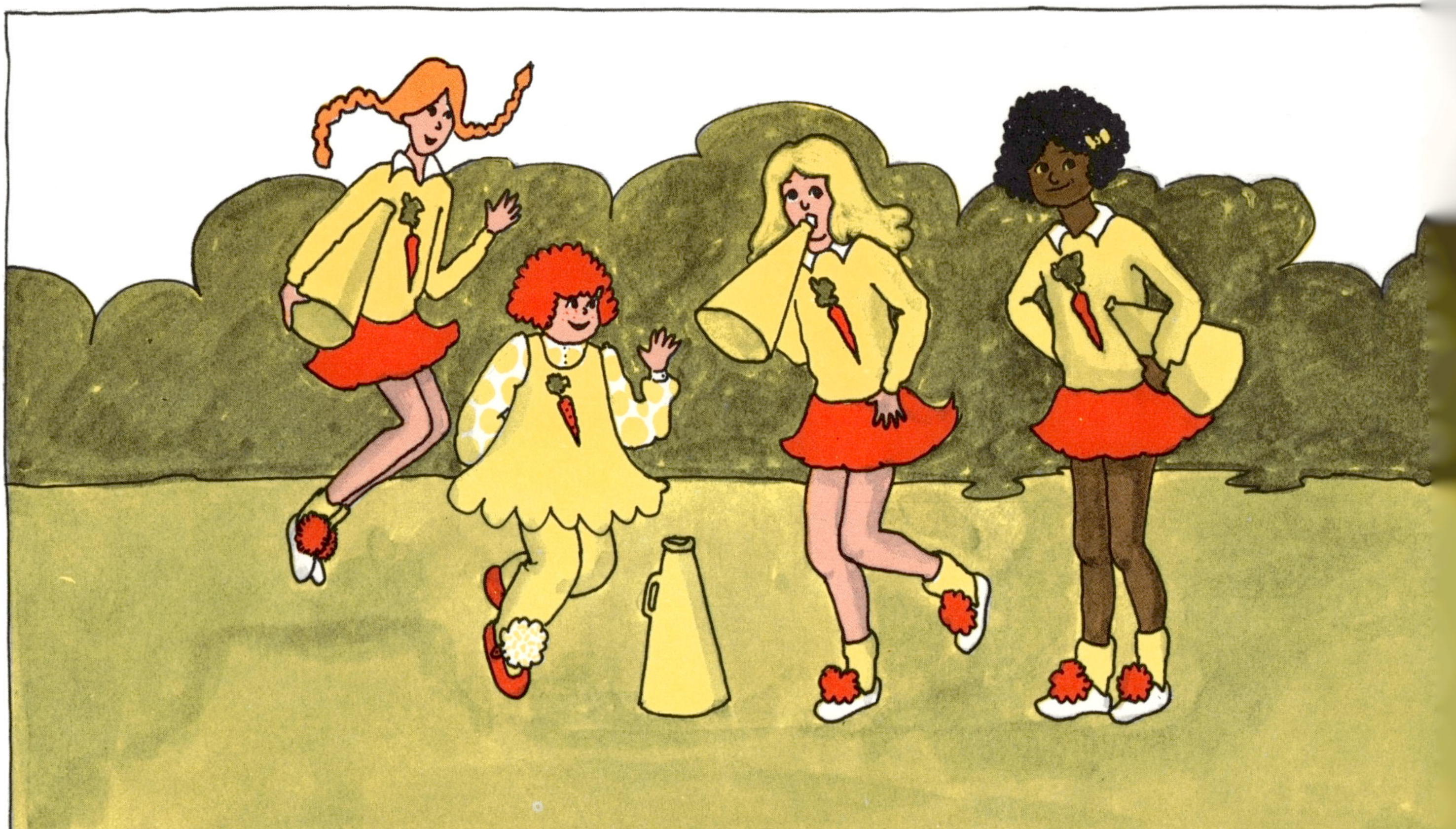

Even if he eats a pound of carrots instead of a pound of cookies, he might still get fat. There are not many calories in carrots, but if the calories are not used up, they may turn into stored-up fat. A football player can eat cookies and never get fat because he uses up the cookies for fuel. But a person watching that football game and eating carrots may get fat.

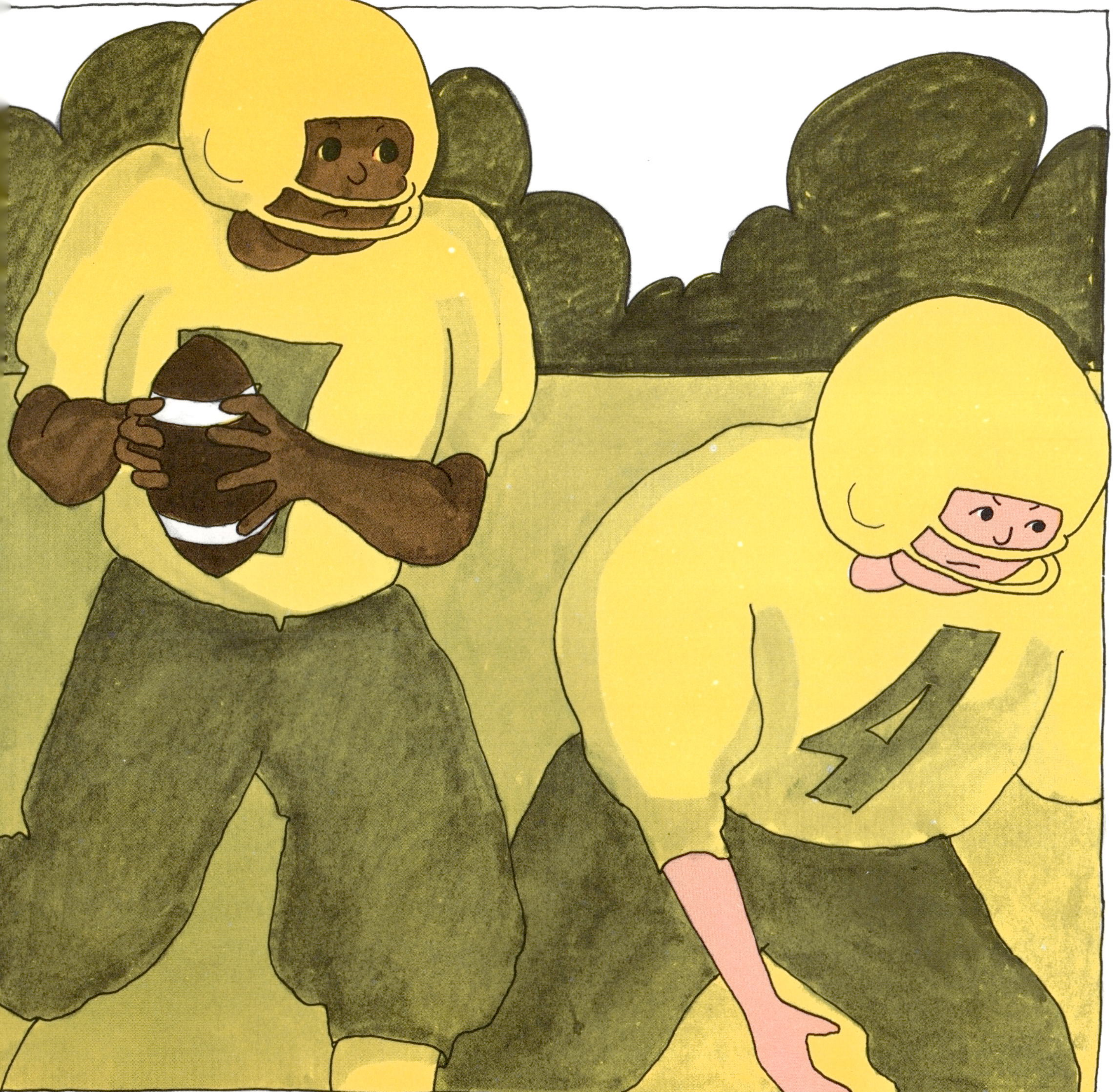

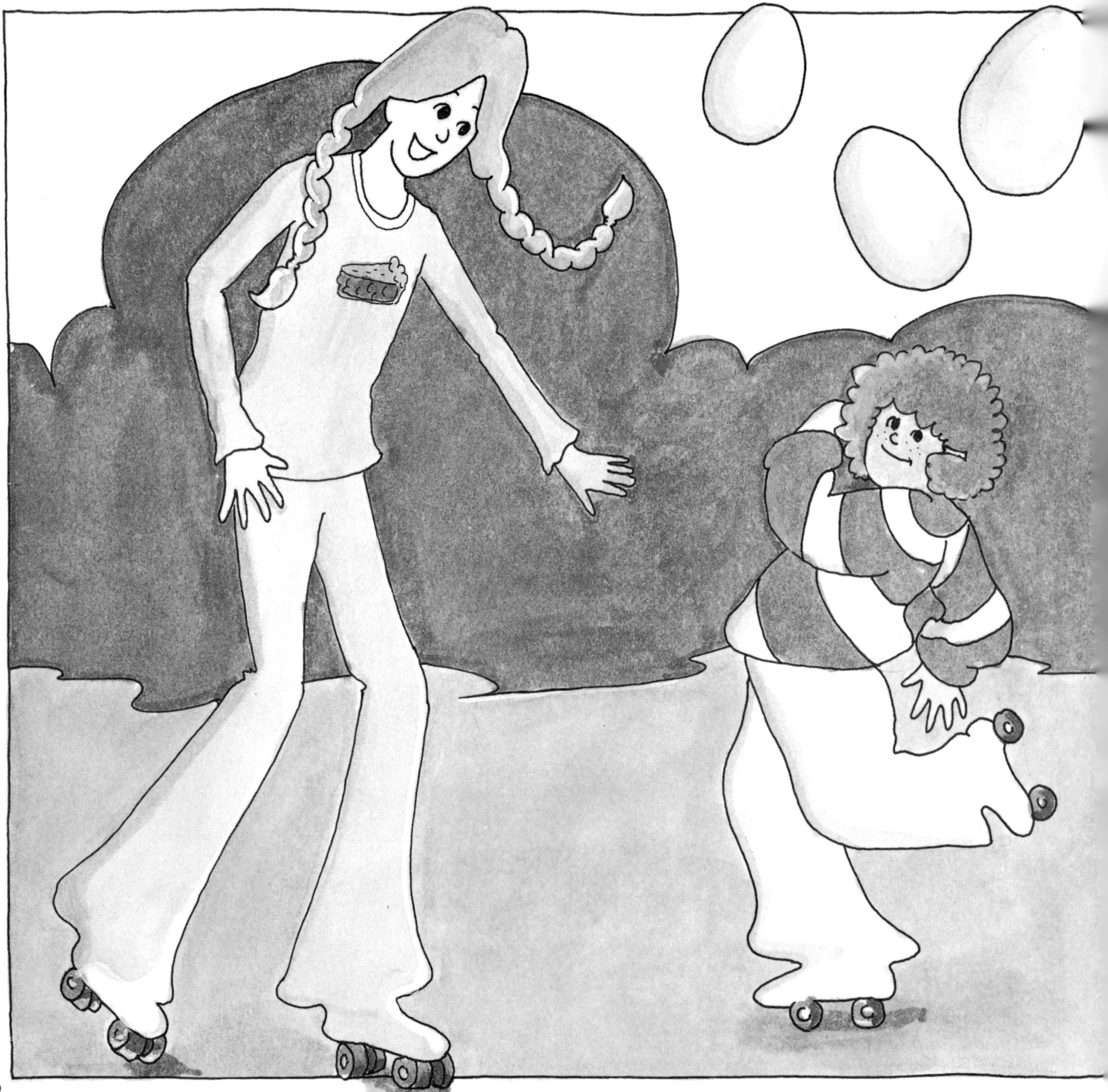

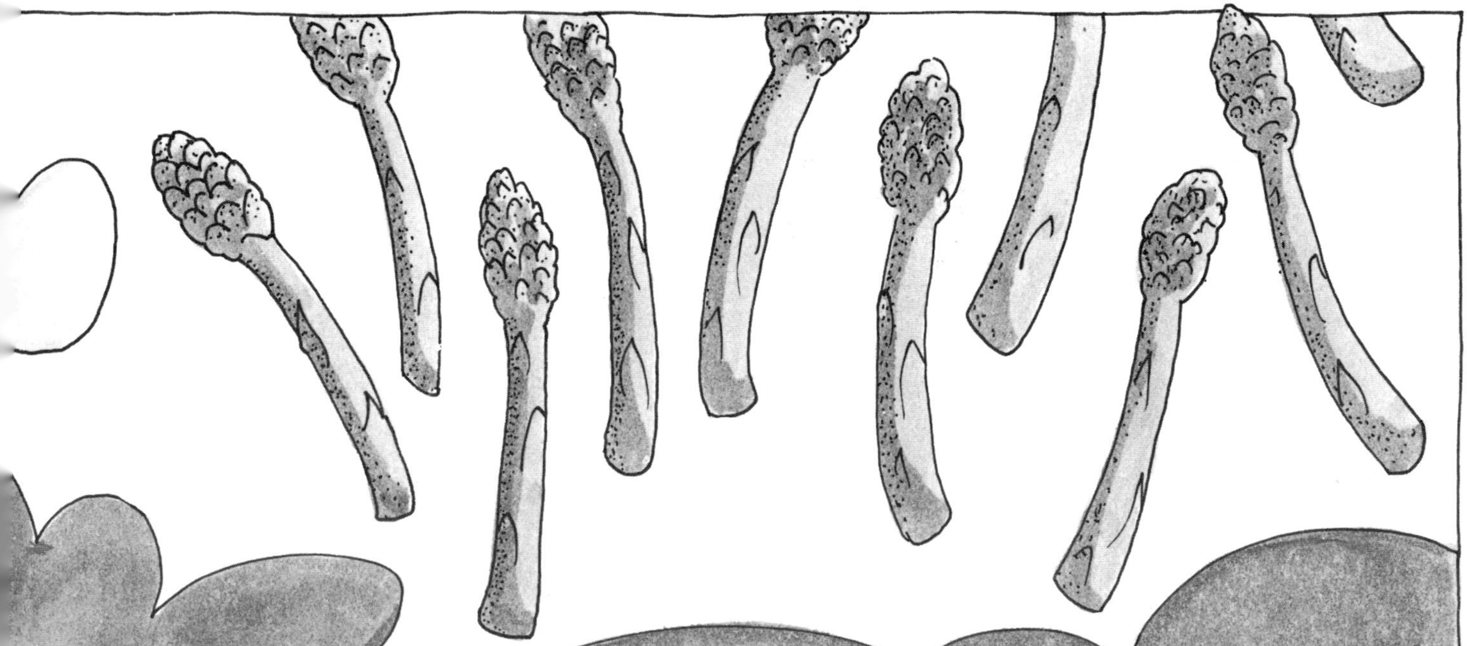

Some foods have more calories than others. The lists show how many calories some foods have. They also tell how you can use up the calories.

Kind of Food	Number of Calories	Kind of Activity per Hour to Use the Calories Up
One huge sirloin steak (8 inches by 5 inches by 2 inches) *or* 120 spears of asparagus	500	bicycling
$9\frac{1}{2}$ boiled eggs *or* 3 plain waffles	650	roller skating

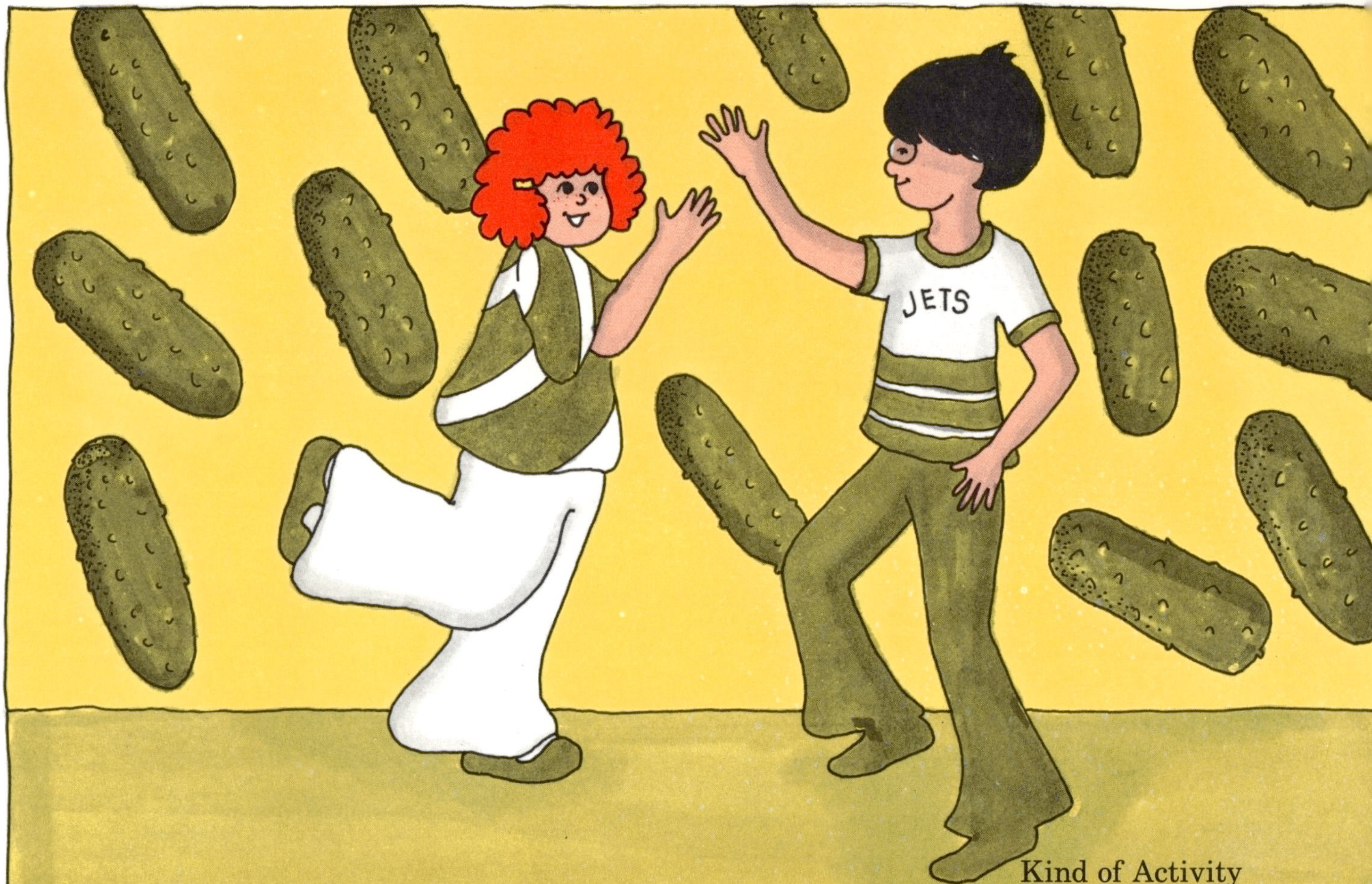

Kind of Food	Number of Calories	Kind of Activity per Hour to Use the Calories Up
A medium-sized slice of apple pie *or* 10 five-inch cantaloupes	377	Ping-Pong
8 squares of cheese ravioli with sauce *or* 66 four-inch-long dill pickles	724	dancing fast

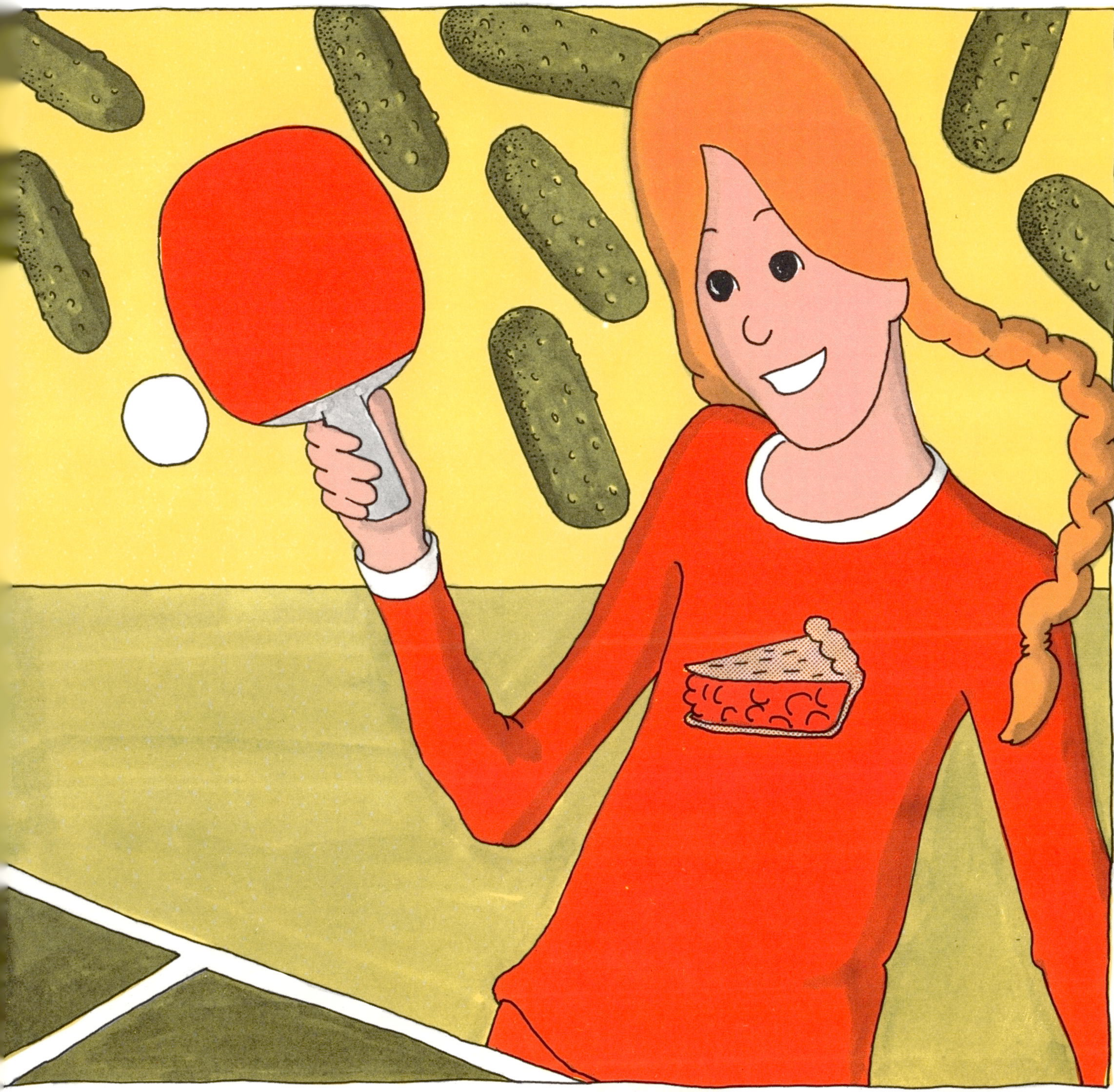

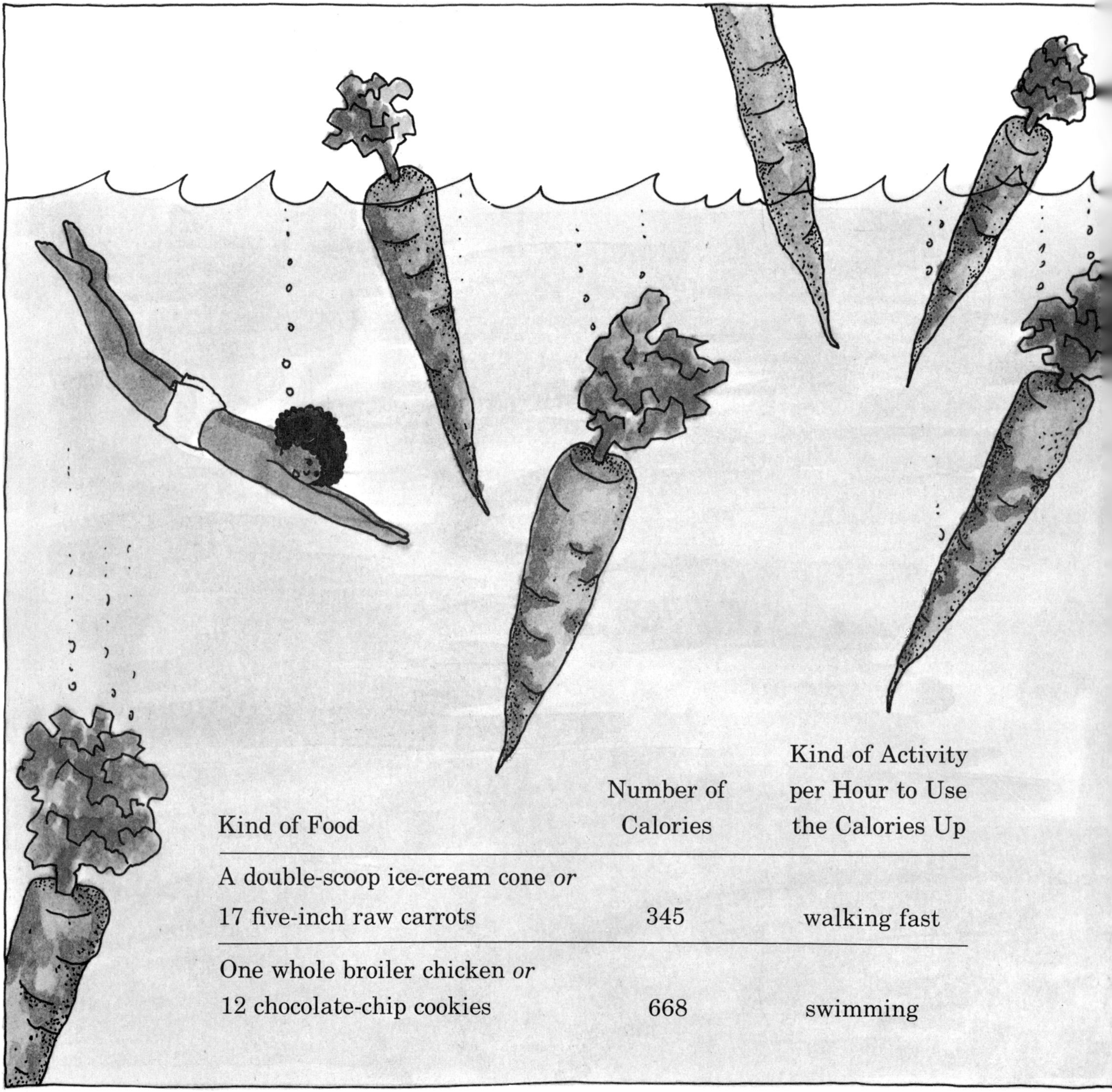

Kind of Food	Number of Calories	Kind of Activity per Hour to Use the Calories Up
A double-scoop ice-cream cone *or* 17 five-inch raw carrots	345	walking fast
One whole broiler chicken *or* 12 chocolate-chip cookies	668	swimming

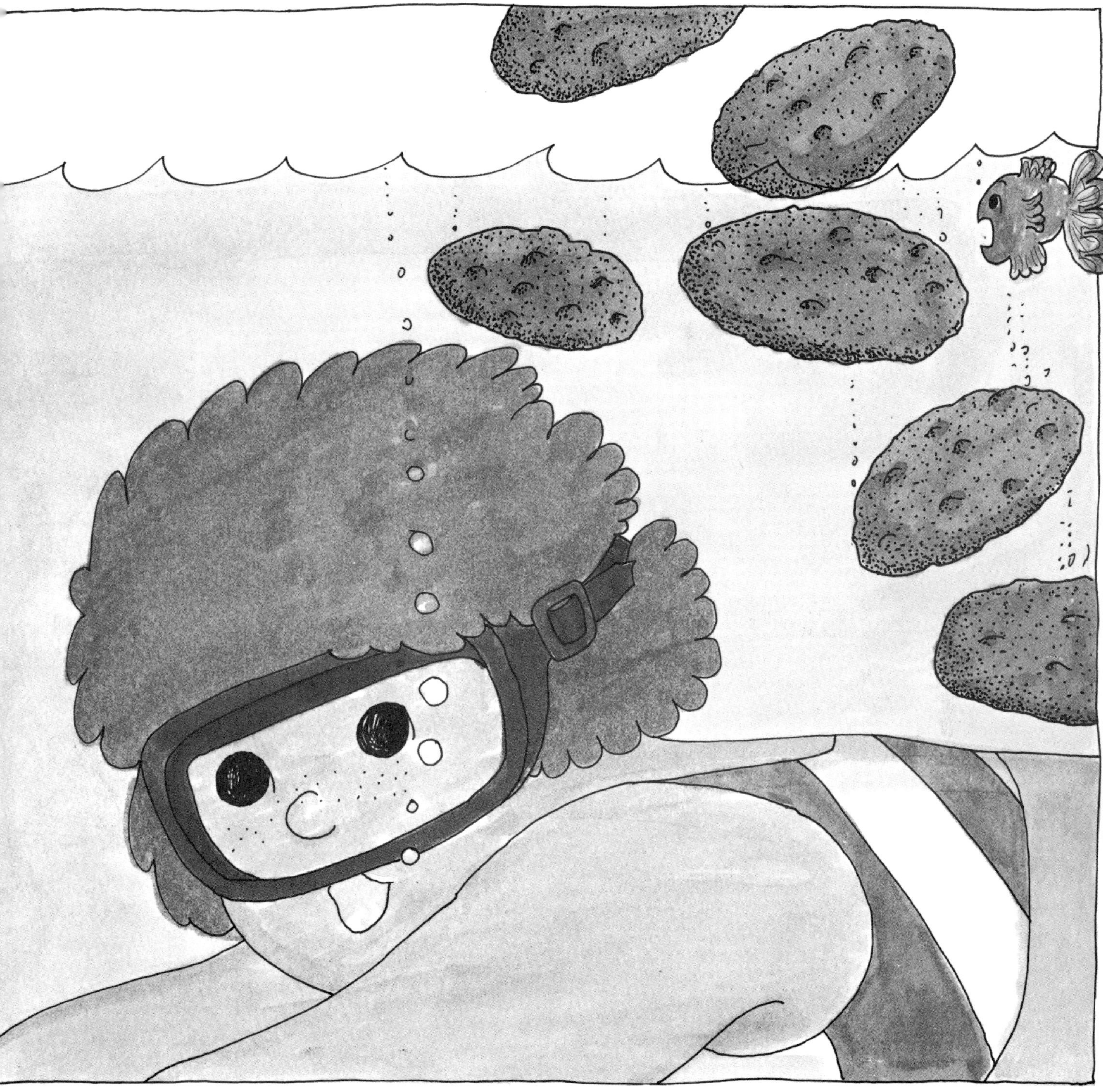

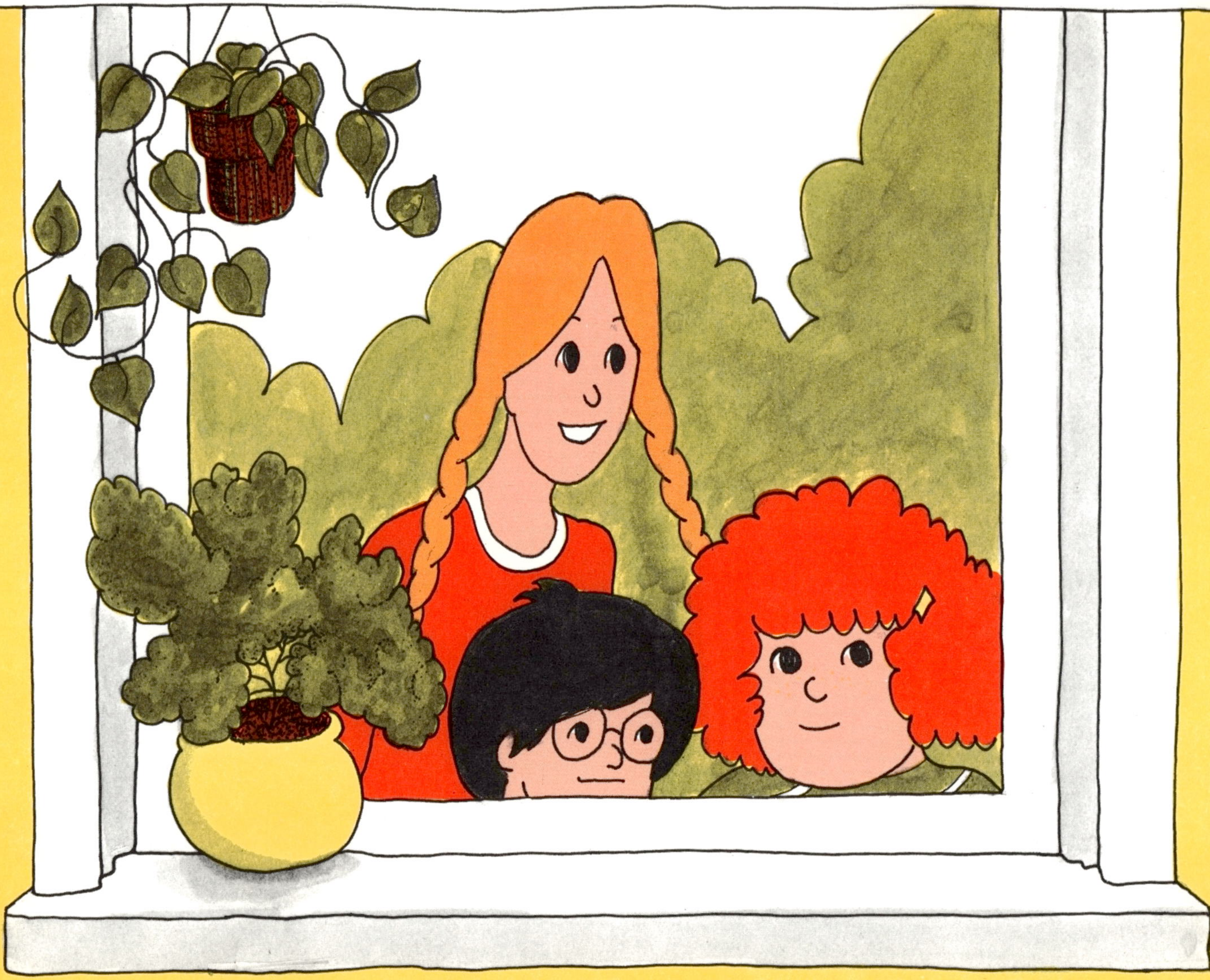

A skinny person may get fatter if he eats foods with a lot of calories. But if he has high metabolism, he won't get much fatter. He uses up the food that he eats.

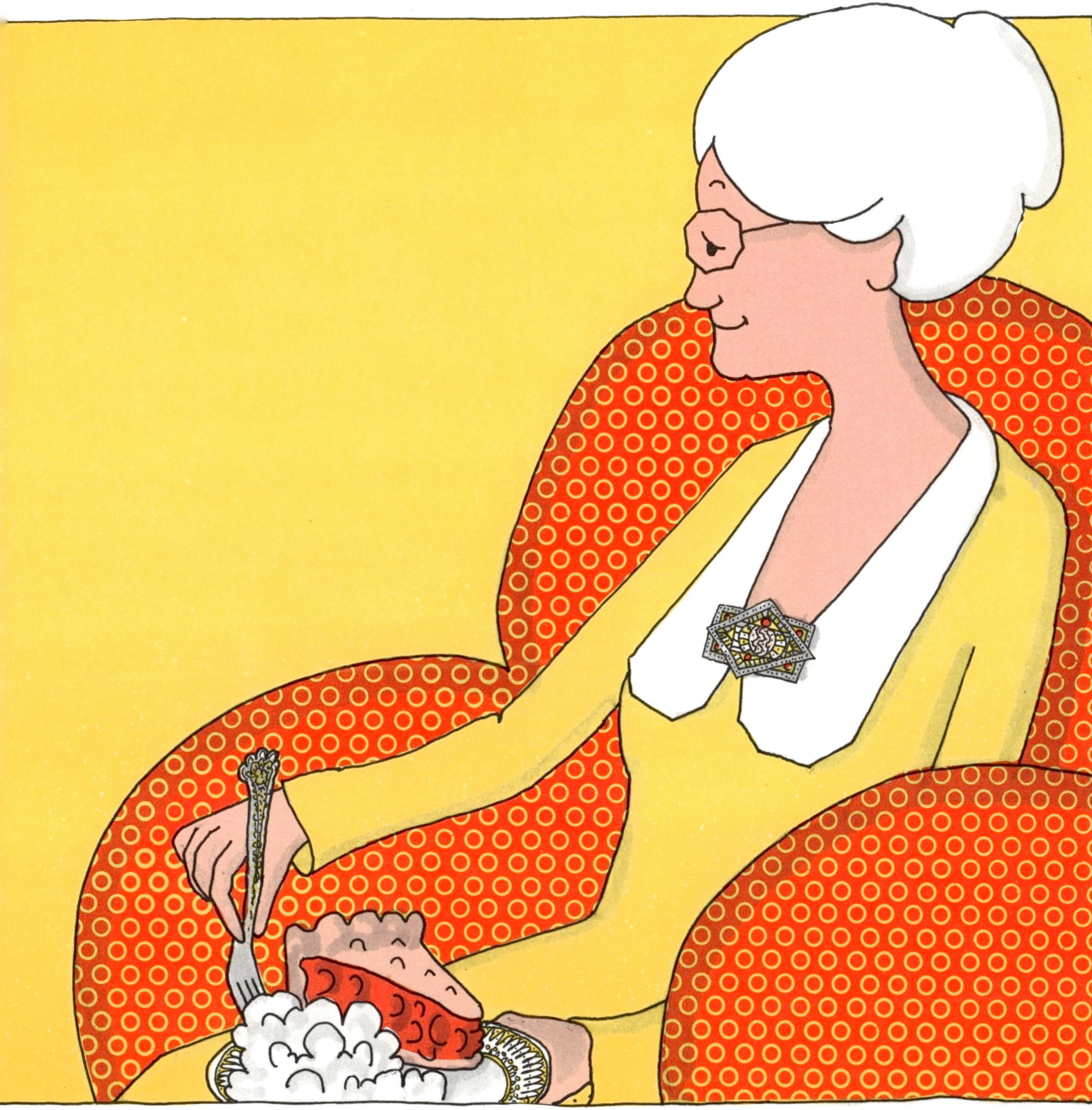

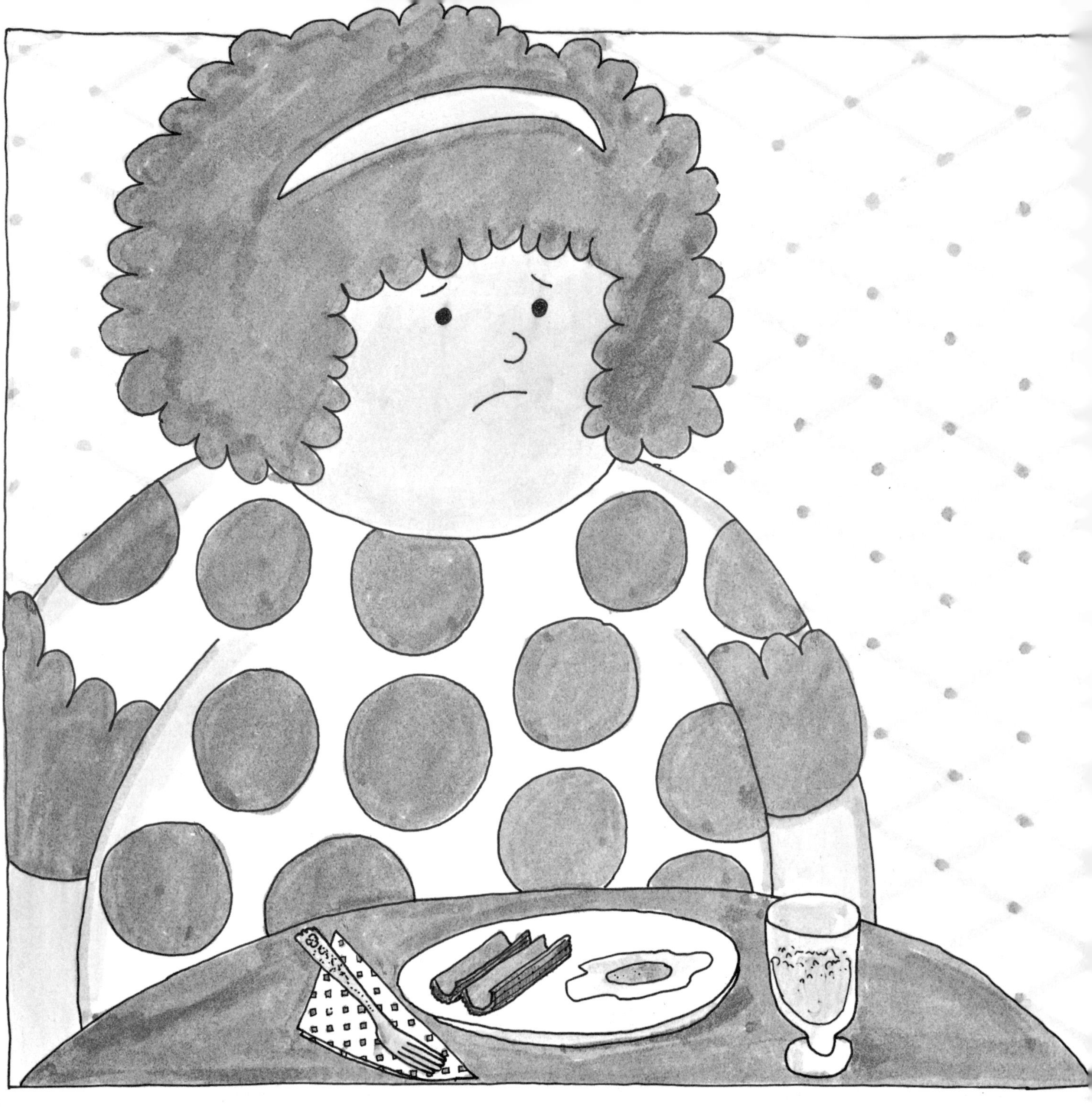

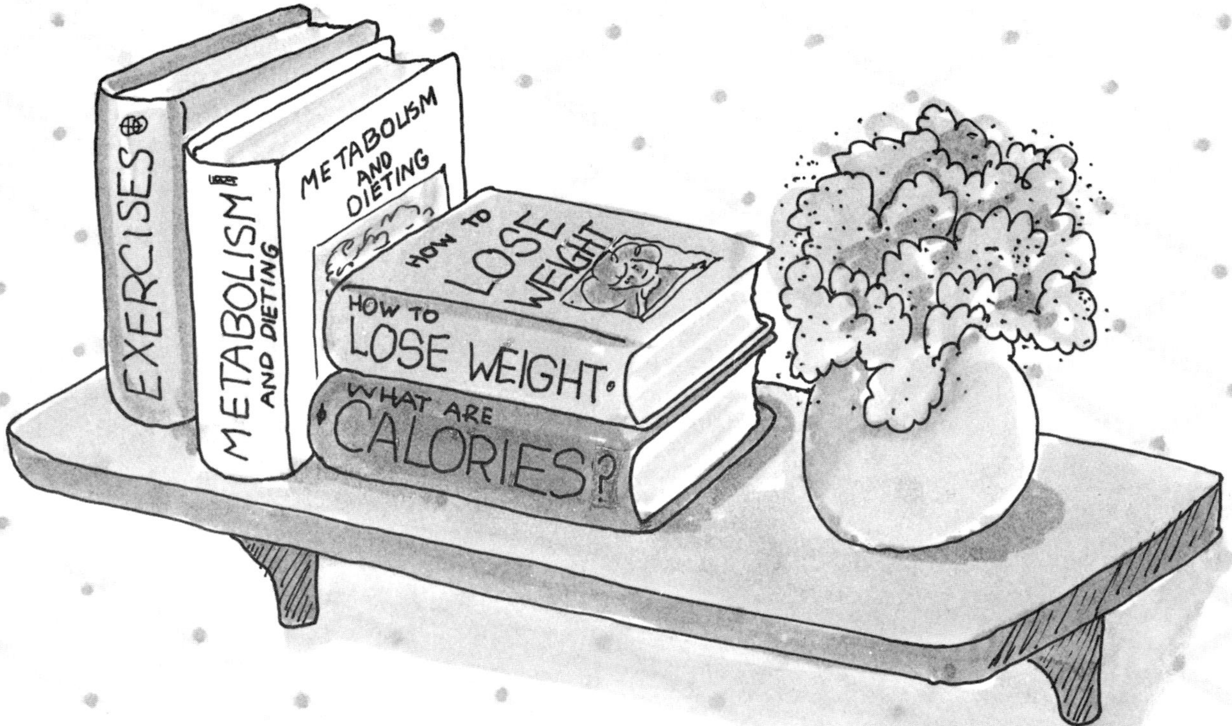

A fat person who wants to get thinner must eat less. And he must not eat foods that have a lot of calories in them. If he has low metabolism, a fat person may never get much thinner. He just doesn't use up the food that he eats. Most fat people can be thinner. They must eat less.

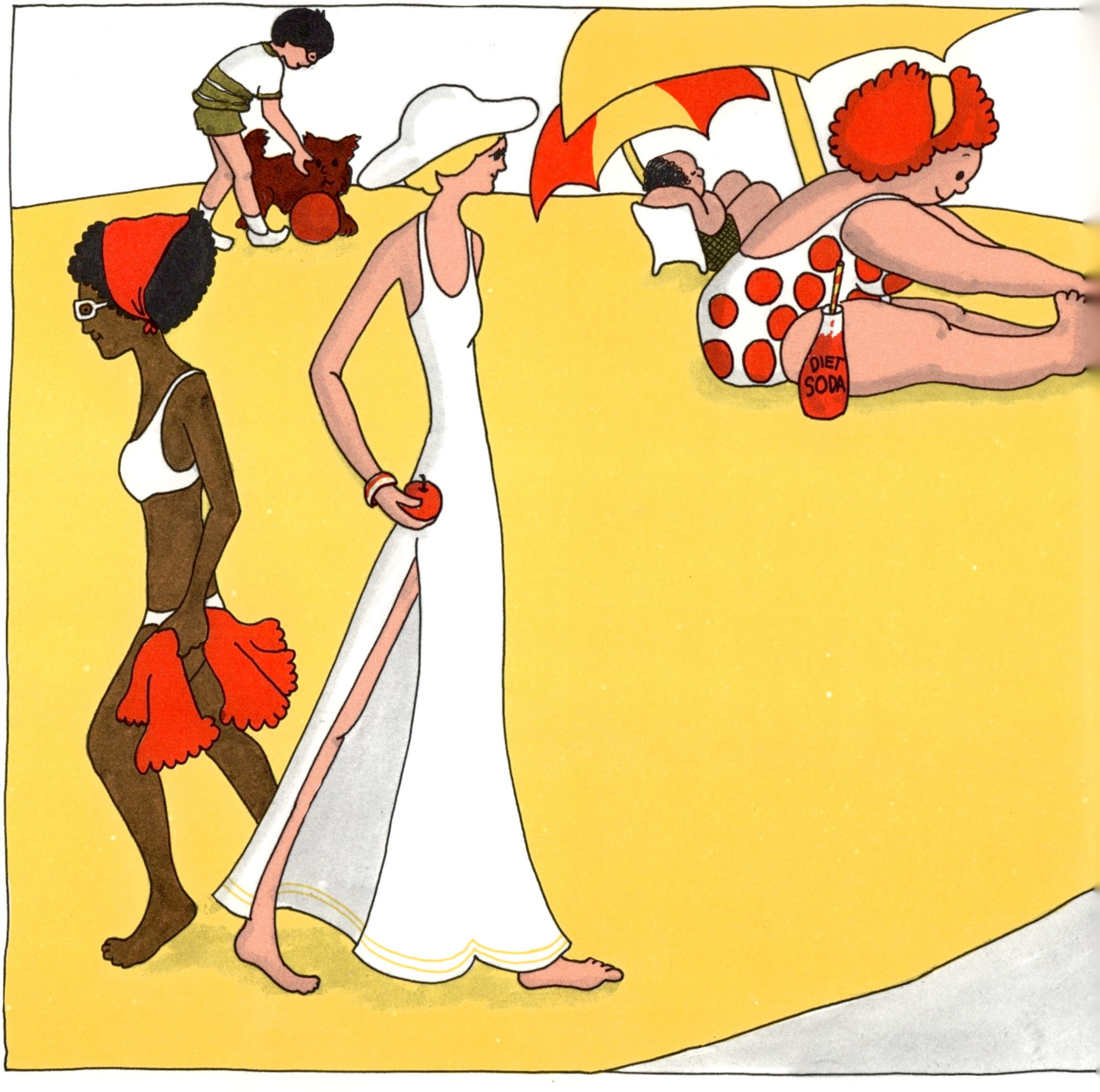
DIET
SODA

People are different. Some people are tall, others are short. Some have big long noses, others have short small ones. Some people are fat, other people are skinny.

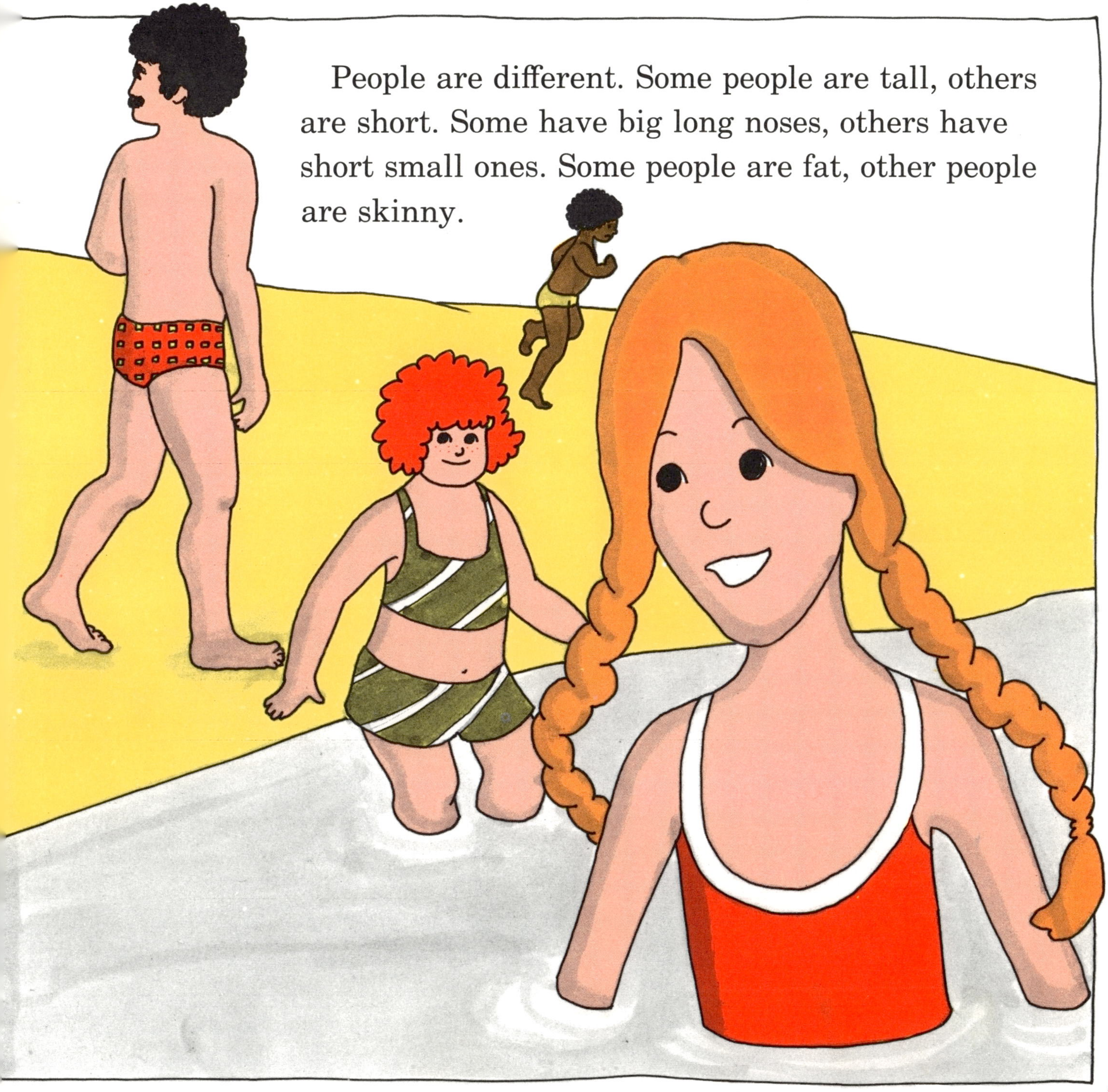

ABOUT THE AUTHOR

Philip Balestrino was a fat child because he ate too many goodies. Now, as an adult, he is of average weight but he still has to watch what he eats. Vanilla ice cream is his favorite fattening food.

Mr. Balestrino lives in Greenwich Village and teaches speech communication at Manhattan Community College. For exercise he walks and bicycles all over New York City, and he burns up lots of calories moving furniture in his Village antiques shop.

ABOUT THE ILLUSTRATOR

Pam Makie studied art at Mohawk Valley Community College in Utica, New York, and at the School of Visual Arts and Cooper Union in New York City. She now lives in New York City, where she is a partner in a graphic design firm. Miss Makie spends much of her time studying comparative philosophy, religion, and psychoanalytical material. She has also taught art to children at a school in New York City.